DOCTOR AND PATIENT

ADRIENNE VON SPEYR

Doctor and Patient

~

Translated by
Frank Nitsche-Robinson

IGNATIUS PRESS SAN FRANCISCO

Original German edition:
Arzt und Patient

Front cover medical symbol from iStock images

Cover design by Roxanne Mei Lum

ISBN 978-1-62164-356-2 (PB)
ISBN 978-1-64229-236-7 (eBook)
Library of Congress Control Number 2024950417
Printed in the United States of America ♾

CONTENTS

FOREWORD

Stephen E. Doran, M.D.[1]

At first blush, *Doctor and Patient* appears to be a memoir of sorts, narrating the various stages of Adrienne von Speyr's medical career. But it is much more important than that. Adrienne is better known for her mystical writings than she is for her career as a physician. Yet she was both: Adrienne the physician and Adrienne the mystic. Were they the same person? The religious skeptic would say no and promote a false dichotomy between faith and reason or mysticism and pragmatism. *Doctor and Patient* dispels this myth.

Adrienne was born in 1902 and raised in an upper-class family in Protestant Switzerland. When she was only six years old, she had what she later believed to be a mystical encounter with Saint Ignatius of Loyola, and when she was fifteen, the Blessed Virgin Mary appeared to her surrounded by angels and saints, including Ignatius. Von Balthasar notes that upon her conversion to Catholicism in 1940, "a veritable cataract

[1] Dr. Stephen E. Doran is a board-certified neurosurgeon, an ordained permanent deacon, and a bioethicist for the Archdiocese of Omaha, Nebraska. His writings in bioethics, neurosurgery, and gene therapy for brain disorders have been widely published in media outlets, textbooks, and academic journals. He is the author of *To Die Well: A Catholic Neurosurgeon's Guide to the End of Life* (Ignatius Press, 2023).

of mystical graces poured over Adrienne in a seemingly chaotic storm that whirled her in all directions at once."[2] He goes on to say, "The theory of mysticism that Adrienne formulated culminates in the one statement: Mysticism is a particular mission, a particular service to the Church that can only be properly carried out in a continual and complete movement away from oneself."[3] Adrienne the mystic and Adrienne the physician drank from the same well of selflessness. She was a tireless advocate for the poor, treating many of them without charge. According to von Balthasar, she saw between sixty and eighty patients per day.[4] She had a particular heart for unwed mothers, and thousands of abortions were prevented under her care.

The physician's worldview is the fundamental basis for the relationship between patient and physician. This worldview influences all the actions of the physician, including the personal relationship with a patient, the diagnosis of an illness, the remedies applied. As Adrienne says, "It is everything; everything must conform to it and has legitimacy insomuch as it can be integrated into it."[5] For Adrienne, her worldview was rooted in the truth of Christ. "Every truth is somehow participation, but participation in God is the highest truth."[6] There was no artificial separation between

[2] Hans Urs von Balthasar, *First Glance at Adrienne von Speyr*, 2nd ed. (Ignatius Press, 2017), 33.

[3] *First Glance*, 36.

[4] *First Glance*, 33.

[5] Chapter IV, p. 87.

[6] Chapter III, p. 74.

faith and reason. Yet at the same time, there is a tension between the two, and as she says, a good dose of humility is necessary to see the harmony between science and Christianity. The individual must assume the responsibility of integrating what seems to be disparate.

When reason is bracketed from faith, the consequence is the depersonalization of medicine. A patient is no longer seen as a person; he is an illness. He becomes dismembered. The pressures of efficiency trump personal intimacy between doctor and patient. The mutual relationship between doctor and patient that should be present requires the physician to come to terms with himself, and only then can he reach maturity. This process requires stillness and silence.[7] It is probably self-apparent that when medicine is depersonalized, the patient suffers. However, the person of the *physician* will also atrophy if he neglects the person in front of him. Technical skills may persist, but he is reduced from an instrument of healing to a technician. As von Speyr writes, "In the end, he would only see the disease, no longer the sick person who suffers it, or the sick person as a necessary evil. He would prefer to have the disease in front of himself in its purest form; the person would only be the cause of its occurrence."[8] This is the heart of the problem with medicine, both now and in Adrienne's time. Death has become medicalized: illness and death are the enemy,

[7] Chapter II, p. 49.
[8] Chapter III, p. 67.

and modern technologies are the weapons to defeat them. In the battle against death, the patient is often reduced to an interested bystander whose humanity and personhood are largely ignored.

Despite the wild successes of new and emerging therapies, patient satisfaction is plummeting. Why? There is no shortage of scapegoats. Health care staff are stretched thin beyond human capacities. Insurance companies reap record profits while patients are denied care. Physician burnout is fueled by burdensome regulations, unrealistic patient expectations, excessive workload, and a host of other factors. The natural consequence of these pressures is a sense of alienation for both patients and providers. Does *Doctor and Patient* provide a quick fix? Of course not. The problems of today are not much different from those of Adrienne's day, and they appear insurmountable, at least on the macro level. However, on the micro level, the one-on-one relationship between doctor and patient can be salvaged. The depersonalization of medicine can be defeated by a worldview that does not hold faith at arm's length. Rooted in the truth of Jesus Christ, the pragmatic and the mystic can, and must, coexist. There is no artificial separation between them.

EDITOR'S PREFACE

As her autobiography shows, already during her medical studies, Adrienne von Speyr was consistently concerned with questions of medical ethics, and at times she even made her decisions in this regard known in a spectacular fashion. During the years of her intensive medical practice, this interest deepened more and more; her intention to write a work on the subject is fully corroborated in its seriousness by very numerous notes—often with only keywords of topics to cover. The grand plan was not carried out, many topics that were to be covered (e.g., death and euthanasia, questions of pastoral medicine, but also seemingly purely practical problems such as that of health insurance and its effects on the behavior of doctor and patient) were not developed. On a few occasions, Adrienne resorted to the narrative form, but after a few pages the at times vivid descriptions break off. There are titles such as: "The first day in the hospital", "The nurse", "The doctor, his youth, and his death".

Of the pieces offered here, all were dictated to the undersigned, except for two, which she submitted for printing: the review of Tournier's book appeared in the *Schweizer Rundschau*, July 1944; the essay "Befruchtende Literatur" (Stimulating literature), under the title "Vom lesenden Arzt" (The reading physician), appeared in the *Festschrift for Fritz Ernst*, Zurich, 1949.

A selection from the handwritten notes on the unfinished work is added to this booklet as a supplement.

However rich this work would have been if it had been completed, the focal questions around which Adrienne's thinking revolves are certainly touched upon in the fragments presented here: the holistically human, responsible introduction of the medical student to his subject, the likewise holistically human, correct behavior of the practicing doctor toward his patients, and finally the comprehensive problem of medical truth as it presents itself in the doctor's knowledge, on the one hand, and in the sick person's experience, on the other hand. The mutual limits of these can only be transcended in the opening to the divine truth—and what is accessible to us of it in Jesus Christ.

The fragments presented here, as well as another booklet with practical instructions for acquaintance, engagement, and marriage (*Christiane*), show how much Adrienne von Speyr realistically cared for the people entrusted to her, and she constantly struggled to mediate between her numerous worldly responsibilities and the abundance of her spiritual insights, to which her scriptural commentaries and other religious works bear witness.

Hans Urs von Balthasar

I
MEDICAL STUDIES

1. The Beginnings

Present and Future

The student who begins his medical studies has a certain image of what he is aiming for. For him, this image lies in the future: in the time when he will be working as a doctor. Most of the time, a certain aspect is at the forefront of his interest: science, helping others, or even shaping his own life as a doctor. He imagines what he will have time for: his patients, but also other things that interest him. It is out of love for this outline of his future that he begins his studies.

But it should be pointed out to him that there is no gap between his present and his future. Everything he undertakes now as a student already belongs to the image he sees as the future; indeed he must—retroactively, as it were—already be shaped by this image. Both the present and the future must mutually influence each other and adapt to each other. Into this developing entity he assimilates himself from the very beginning. He cannot study with only one part of his personality, his mental powers, for example, and ignore all other aspects for the time being. A whole person should devote himself to a whole study in order to shape a whole life.

First Personal Attitude Adjustment

The focus on wholeness requires a certain attitude toward oneself from the outset, which then also influences the attitude toward the material to be learned and—in the clinical semesters—toward patients and colleagues. Even at this early stage, the relationship to fellow students and other people must be such that the later transition into the circle of patients and colleagues can take place organically. He who begins his studies should from the very beginning want to be the person he envisions to be in practice at the end of his studies. He must not, for example, pursue his studies so egotistically and exclusively that everything else, above all, the cultivation of humanity, appears secondary to him, as if only one thing were important now, to "cram"; everything else will be dealt with later. Already at this stage he owes it to himself to make his existence harmonious and balanced.

There will always be some material in his studies that appeals to him and some that does not. Much will seem like filler to him, but it is in the curriculum; he must acquire it. Perhaps he does not understand the disposition of this curriculum, but that is irrelevant. He is not one of those who have to design it, but one of those who have to follow it and acquire what is prescribed. This, first and foremost, requires discipline and obedience: this particular exam is mandatory, I have to pass it. Of course we have our preferences, but one must not neglect the rest of the program out of defiance and knowing better. The beginner sees things from below: his perspective can be skewed, even wrong. A good dose of humility is needed here. Students usually act as if they are superior to everything. Instead, they should recognize the work of those who created the curriculum. Even if someone were convinced that something was wrong or superfluous, he should submit to what has been given to him. Perhaps he will later be able to make an argument for what he thinks he knows better. First he must mature in what he does not understand now.

On the other hand, medicine is not the absolute, and so there is also the converse demand: to integrate what presents itself into one's own worldview, especially if this worldview is Christian, Catholic. This, of course, primarily requires that one knows what it means to be Catholic. At the beginning of the studies, the natural sciences have the upper hand; they must somehow be compatible with Christianity. Naturally, the student cannot expect the harmony between science and Christianity to be evident everywhere. But he should not separate the two in his mind as if there were no relationship at all, but should try to understand as much as possible of this relationship. Wherein does the truth lie, wherein the limit of the proposition that man is descended from apes? It will certainly not be possible to abolish the "superior" discussions among students, but the individual should have enough responsibility to try personally to integrate what seems disparate. Otherwise everything will suddenly seem empty and hollow for him.

The material itself stimulates the learner's sense of responsibility and thus deepens his central worldview. Humility in study promotes his Christian humility. It also protects him from arrogance for the very reason that everything he has learned is ultimately based on the achievements of others. One learns things that did not present themselves, but had to be considered and researched by others before they could be presented to him on a platter. Every doctor owes a debt of gratitude to the researchers who have worked before him, which is why no community of pride should develop among doctors, professors, and students. They are all part of a tradition that they did not create, but merely continue.

In the lower semesters, the subject matter makes few direct references to God; nevertheless, the student should integrate science and religion and, to that end, seek to clarify his worldview: to acquire as much philosophy and theology as is necessary for sound pastoral medicine. He should strengthen the awareness within himself that not everything can be dissected spiritually or literally. Above all, he should not think that he can bring about a quick synthesis. If a man seeks God in every insect, he will become a superficial pantheist, or his religious feeling will become dull and everything will ultimately disgust him. It should be enough for him if a certain light emanating from the big picture, a guideline, shines on his daily work.

Encounter with the Body

When the student begins to dissect the human body, it takes on an unreal quality as a result of having been prepared to such a degree. It takes a downright effort to remember that these limbs, which may have been lying in a formalin solution for years and are dark and tanned, belonged to a living person. Moreover, these corpses are without viscera. Only occasionally is work done on a fresh corpse so as to become familiar with the position of the organs.

The person lies before you, dissected into his bones and muscles, so much so that you only perceive the pieces you have under your fingers and whose causalities you can overlook. One corpse may be shared among twenty students, and the limb that each one of them receives must be separated from the whole as soon as possible so that he can begin his work. The body lying on the table is removed piece by piece, the integrity of this body, even the relationship of this once living human being to God, recedes into an intangible distance. The student does not possess the synthetic power to resist such a dissection of reality without further ado. He is completely occupied with memorizing the correct designation for each nerve, etc. Now he is in even more urgent need of a firm worldview than before in order not to lose touch with God even outside of working hours.

At the same time, he pursues constructive-synthetic physiology and physiological chemistry in order to understand the functioning of the human organism. Both try somehow to build this organism seamlessly from matter to a life. In a way, this, too, has an effect of dissection, because everything starts with the elementary. In anatomy, the human being was dissolved, but now the elements are used to rebuild the equivalent of a human. In the process one gets the feeling that the physiological human is completely different from the anatomical one. The latter is dead and is becoming more and more so. The former, on the other hand, slowly comes to life from the dead. Homunculus! It can be produced in a test tube.

During this time, sexuality almost always becomes a problem for the student. What one learned about it in zoology hardly related to the human experience. Now the human organs become relevant. In physiology, the student is inclined to observe what he has learned, the mechanism of breathing, for instance, on himself. This also leads to the temptation to try out the sexual functions. The girls less so than the young men, who, if they are not in fraternities and have their girls, also explore these things with each other.

During this period, in addition to their studies, they need rest, relaxation, the counterbalance of beauty—music, pictures—something wholesome and fulfilling that tunes the whole person, something that also endures in its beauty and distracts from the constant deconstruction and construction.[1]

The last semesters before the second propaedeutic exam present an actual overload. You started studying to help living people at some point—and now you no longer see people, only individual reactions. And in an atmosphere of the dead at that. After the anatomy lesson, you feel like you stink. All your clothes are full of it. You stink right down to your skin. At this stage it is impossible to engage a student immediately in a religious conversation. You have to let him air out and relax for a day at least . . .

2. The Clinical Studies

Difficult Atmosphere

Now we finally come to the human person. This is what you have been waiting for and what you have endured your first semesters for. The sick person arrives, but surrounded by a crowd of healthy people: nurses, doctors, assistants. But the human atmosphere into which you enter here is in many regards a clouded one: everyone knows that you are only a student, but

[1] If I, Adrienne, imagine that I had already been Catholic at that time—by upbringing, about average Catholic—would I then not have felt a strong resistance to seeing the Body of Christ in a consecrated Host? The "transfigured body", where "body" always brings to mind the dead and the mechanical? And what would a confession have been? A mere dissection of one's consciousness?

to the sick people whom you have to examine you are introduced as a doctor. No sick person is stupid enough to believe that. The real reason for such a distortion of the truth is that the patient is not taken seriously in his humanity.

I was lucky enough to have a teacher[2] who approached every patient who came into the lecture hall in an entirely personal manner. He approached the patient and told him that it would not be easy for him to show himself to the students, but that it was also a benefit for him that he, the professor, would take care of his case personally. And whenever possible, he himself did, in fact, operate on the patient. Through his conversation with the patient, which all those around could overhear, he initiated a relationship between the patient and the students. If a case was hopeless, he said goodbye to the patient, who was led out, and discussed the rest with the students alone, but did not fail to visit the patient again afterward, explain his condition, and prepare him for death in his own way. He always knew how far he could go with the disclosure. He never said: "You will be fine" if he knew that this was not the case.

Other doctors didn't seem to care at all about the patient's personality. For them, the person brought into the room was a "case". This was the essential, the true thing; the person behind it seemed almost like a lie,

[2] Prof. Dr. Gerhard Hotz. Cf. Adrienne von Speyr, *My Early Years*, trans. Mary Emily Hamilton and Dennis D. Martin (Ignatius Press, 1995), 329–94.

and in the process you yourself felt like an even bigger lie. And a person who is forgotten as such in the lecture hall is also of no further concern to the doctor afterward. If there is a risk of the patient dying in the lecture hall, he is removed in due time. Death in the lecture hall is frowned upon. However, if an intimate procedure is to be carried out, it is done in the lecture hall. Actually, it would not even be necessary for the entire audience to be present. In the ward there can also be difficult cases, catheterization, for example. The nurse isn't able to do it and calls in the doctor. He in turn calls in a few students: "Come along, there's something entertaining going on! . . ."

There are, of course, caring nurses in the hospitals who are trying to make up for the damage done. A Penelope job! After the doctor's rounds, they mend what will surely be torn again tomorrow or the day after.

Thus the student can initially be very disappointed with the human atmosphere in the hospital. Other things appeal to him, even inspire him: he now sees how smooth the transitions are from anatomy to pathology, how quickly he can find his way around if he has previous knowledge. In the beginning, it all does not seem difficult because he is presented with clear, transparent cases and has the feeling that he has already mastered the essentials with a number of diagnoses that he can make from what he has learned.

But from the second semester onward, the student is bombarded with such a confusing abundance of information that he is in danger of getting completely lost. He has the feeling of a small section of the whole being assigned to him, because he doesn't yet have an overview of the whole. He is sent to the wards to examine, but this is inconvenient for the nurses, the patient is disgruntled because he has already been examined many times by others. The student realizes that social issues, questions of insurance, care, and poverty play an important role for many. It is also confusing that there are patients wrestling with death lying next to others who have almost no signs of illness; the interest in either of them, however, appears to be the same, whether they die today or will be discharged tomorrow. No one accompanies the dying into their death. The hospital priest is only called when the patient is lost. The entire operation is mechanized.

The student wants to break through the all-dominating impersonality; he should at least try. Perhaps he can strike up a conversation, or perhaps he can bring the patients small gifts. He feels that he must not only take, but should also give something.

The Hospital Hierarchy

Medical responsibility in a hospital is precisely distributed only in theory. The ultimate responsibility lies with the senior physician in the department; the assistant stands between him and the students. Authorizations are for the most part unclear. The senior physician does not know exactly what his assistants can do: for certain things he himself has authorization, in others only the boss does, in still others they both do. The assistant also often does not know to what extent he will be supported or overruled, for example, during the senior physician's rounds. Such ambiguity at times leads to the assistant becoming somewhat indifferent or trying to show off personally in order somehow to belittle the senior physician in front of the patients and gain authority himself. Everyone wants to be seen by the patients as the boss.

There is also mistrust among the fellow assistants. The difference in length of service plays a big role: this one arrived a month later than me; he can't do anything yet. If you have already been an assistant for longer, you expect the others to recognize your priority. The entire hierarchy is permeated by a wave of contempt, into which the students are also drawn: they learn to despise the boss a little because he wants so little to do with the patients. In the first semesters you have respect for the professors; in the last semesters you are excessively inundated with inadequacies.

The lack of clarity in the distribution of responsibilities leads to a lack of clarity in behavior toward patients; the uncertainty in the medical field leads to uncertainty in the spiritual and moral field—uncertainty about what one should say to a patient, what he can or cannot bear. One hesitates until he has to be taken out of the hall, and only in extremis are a few honest words spoken.

Of course, one encounters all different kinds of assistants in a hospital; those who are only concerned with the formal execution of their duties, and others who take on a considerable amount of human responsibility toward the patients, who as a result can arrive at diametrically opposed views of a hospital, depending on which room they were in. For the exoneration of the assistants, it must be said that the wards are almost always too large. If someone has sixty patients to look after, with all the back and forth in the hospital, the arrival of relatives, and his own scientific work, he will have little time to deal with individual patients in greater detail.

Everyone is advised to keep as far away as possible from medical cliques and instead focus more on the patients.

Depersonalization of Patients[3]

Every patient comes from an environment that has formed him and that he himself has helped to form. There is the worker who comes from his family and was the authority figure in it. There is the girl who comes from an office that she has chosen herself for her livelihood, however modest her position may be, and outside working hours she shapes her life according to her own taste.

Once they enter a hospital as patients, both of them have to renounce their environment and thus somehow also their personality. Even if the patient does not

[3] In the following, the author describes things that she experienced as a student and perhaps also as a physician; many things will have changed considerably since then.—Ed.

become a mere number, he does become a labeled case. Depending on the label, he is put into this room[4] or that. There are cancer rooms, heart rooms, TB rooms. In the women's hospital, there are rooms for patients before surgery; others according to the expected duration of recovery; in these the patient finds entirely different people from those in the previous room.

The patients, who are deprived of their personal environment and their habits and have thus reached a zero point, are forced to form a kind of community with those present in the room, based more or less on the very thing that is unpleasant for everyone, the illness. But before such a community can begin: no sooner did they arrive, still without their bearings, still without knowing the nurses and doctors, and even less so the eight to ten fellow patients in the room, than they are questioned by a doctor about all the intimacies of their lives. Women, for example, are asked to report whether they have already gone through an abortion or had a sexually transmitted disease; the whole room is listening, including the auxiliary staff who are bringing the coffee or mopping the floor. The one asking the question is himself perhaps only a student who has to take the anamnesis, or a doctor surrounded by students. After the student—a sub-assistant—follows another assistant, who again goes through the same questions in front of the entire room and perhaps crudely brings up things that the first one didn't dare to ask.

[4] The author uses the word *Saal* here, which indicates a rather large room for ten or more patients.—Trans.

And no sooner does the patient say what is embarrassing for him, than he is stripped stark naked in front of everyone. If he is unable to pass water, he is catheterized without further ado. (In such rooms you never meet a sick doctor. Either he can afford first class, or he does the impossible to avoid coming to this hospital).

The patient treated in this way must therefore, after the initial renunciation of his own environment, often while still recovering from that first shock, experience a second: the renunciation of his bodily intimacy. What is left for him to do after this exposure but try to adapt to the atmosphere of the hospital room? After all, the others are exposed to him just as he was to them. The new intimacy that arises here is not exactly uplifting. Occasionally there are individual nurses who are not indifferent and help to improve the atmosphere. But for the time being, the newcomer senses little of this better atmosphere; he still lacks the antennae to grasp it.

After a few days he has settled in, but then he is unexpectedly introduced to the students, a new exposition that is frightening for him, so that when he returns to his room, he finds the intimacy there almost pleasant, the strange camaraderie of people who were tossed together by the coincidence of illness. Of course, it is also possible that the patient presented in the lecture hall, surrendered for the third time, has somehow become curious as a result of what he has already experienced. If he is again treated tactlessly, he goes for a sensation and returns to his room with more or less false reports.

In this way, the patient's renunciation of his own dignity can become final. A lot of people are perverted in hospitals. Not just sexually, but more deeply: they get into a false relationship with their bodies. Shame has been lost, nothing matters. A young girl comes into the room with her innate sense of shame and instinctively covers herself. Then she sees how others don't do it and perhaps gets used to it. The others: "We had to laugh because of you, on the first day!" Everything subtle becomes dulled.

The hospital atmosphere is conducive to sensationalism. Among women, there is a strong sexual manifestation. There can be entire rooms where women only talk about their husband's qualities, his virility, or about their own personal adventures. One person can be enough to infect the entire room. Among men, boasting about their illness is more prevalent. The women praise the men's sexual potency, while the men substitute their sexual potency, of which they cannot make use at the moment, with the potency of the illness. Only from the outside—by doctors, nurses, even the students—could these tendencies be countered.

Unmarried mothers are particularly exposed. They have the right to spend three weeks before the birth in the women's hospital free of charge. In return, they serve as "objects" for the students. They have to make themselves available to them every day. Among them are decent girls who accidentally slipped once. Now they are objects for demonstration and are examined vaginally in front of several students. Finally, they have to give birth in front of an entire auditorium without anyone exchanging a kind word with them. There is a lot of unnecessary and avoidable crudeness here. Better use could be made of anesthesia. In fact, married women should also be used so that the entire burden does not fall on the unmarried mothers. It would be easy to treat the women with reverence and kindness instead of a mental crudeness that threatens to rob the students of all reverence for the human body.

The Student

The student should keep an account of the spiritual state of the patients in the hospital. This state is quite different from that of a person in the doctor's consulting room; it is the state of someone who has been dispossessed in many respects. The body of the patient in the hospital should be worth as much to the student as his own body. As a doctor-to-be, he should train himself to be completely objective. This applies, above all, to the examinations he has to carry out.

Someone, for instance, has the task of inserting his finger into the vagina to feel the uterus. He may tremble in front of the professor and not dare to admit that he feels nothing, but he has a *duty* to examine properly, and to do so until the result is achieved without being distracted by any external factors (e.g., his erotic excitement). Otherwise the patient, who has to subjugate herself to this examination, will be "used up" in vain.

There are others who want too much. They have a limited assignment, and they do more. Out of an urge to master the whole thing as quickly as possible, to show the professors all they can do. Such false zeal also results in the abuse of the female patient. Many students do not even know what an objective assignment is and what obedience is.

The need to "collect" diagnoses usually increases from semester to semester, and this addiction is to blame for the fact that the patient is only seen as a "case", as a puzzle that can be taken apart and put together. Someone then goes from room to room as a junior assistant or before his state exam and looks at people based on his skills: "I can do this one, this one, too, that one I have to study more closely. . ."

When the student takes the patients' anamneses in the hospital, they confide their past to him, naturally their physical past at first, which, however, cannot be completely separated from their mental past. In the course of a morning, he gets to hear a whole series of such confidential confessions. He may not even realize that he is making a selection in the end: the main features of the illness are the material for his diagnosis, the human aspects he discards as one discards the pit or the skin of a fruit. He does not consider that the whole person is ill and should recover as a whole person. But it is precisely this wholeness that he will have to take into account as a practicing doctor in the future.

One could point out here the relationship between medical diagnosis and sacramental confession. When someone has laid out his sins in confession, absolution restores to him the wholeness of his personality. This also includes the "skin". This is precisely what does not usually happen in the hospital. By omitting the holistic view, the patient is seduced into seeing himself as just a "case". This makes him even more alienated from his family, his environment, and his work; he can become fanatical about his illness. What is interesting about it has been shown to him, and now he becomes addicted to making it even more interesting. In the hospital, patients like to exaggerate. And foolishly, telling him he has a rare liver disease or the very disease that is currently the subject of intensive research is considered doing the patient a favor. Subsequently it is not uncommon for him to exaggerate the whole thing to such an extent that his illness becomes his actual purpose in life. In the eyes of his family, he becomes the bearer of his illness. When discharged from hospital, readjustment at home is difficult anyway. It is made even more difficult if he has focused entirely on himself in hospital and has thus become an egoist. Now he is offended if his family is not as interested in the illness he had as the other patients in the hospital, who boost each other in overemphasizing the seriousness of their ailment.

II

PRACTICE

1. Setup

To open a practice, the young doctor needs rooms, equipment, and instruments. As he contemplates their purchase, he realizes the magnitude of the change. In a sense, he somehow migrates from the homely familiarity of the clinic into the "enemy camp". First of all, he no longer has his boss behind him, who covers for potential mistakes. In addition, he will no longer have the wealth of auxiliaries provided by the hospital to make precise, scientific diagnoses. If you visit a sick person at home, it is very often not possible to carry out exact examinations in the most recent sense. Therefore a city doctor does right to admit a patient that requires a more subtle diagnosis to a hospital and only make a tentative diagnosis himself. To the young scientist in the clinic, who measures everything by the yardstick of accuracy, he thereby proves his incompetence; the assistant loves to smile about the city doctor, of whose true ability he cannot form a picture after his merely tentative diagnosis. The health insurance companies, on the other hand, require the doctor to make a precise diagnosis. It will usually be the correct one; but in some cases, he cannot help but write "suspected" or make some related diagnosis.

The young doctor setting up his practice becomes cognizant of all this. He realizes that he is transitioning into the camp of the "approximate". He cannot acquire all the expensive equipment of the clinic and is therefore unable to use all of the refined methods. With the purchase of one thing, he will forego another one, if his means are limited. He is somehow losing the ground under his feet. Examinations that were commonplace for him in the hospital he will now have to forego. Consequently his responsibility changes. It increases because he now has to make decisions on his own without backing. It changes because henceforth he has to find solutions based on different considerations.

New Relationship with the Patient

When the first patient arrives, the young doctor realizes how different his situation is. In the hospital, much longer times were expected before a diagnosis and decision could be made. There was a maximum number of examinations, and for each new one the results of the previous ones could be used. Everything needed for a blood transfusion, for instance, was available in the emergency ward. In a private practice consultation, these advantages are lost: the doctor has to arrive at the greatest possible clarity in a minimum of time and with a minimum of examinations, if only because he is going to discharge the patient into an environment where the progress of his condition cannot be monitored in the same way as in the hospital. He must discharge the patient with instructions that will not become obsolete shortly after, due to new developments. In the clinic, if you are unsure, you can always wait for further results; here you have to decide, act, and give instructions immediately. There the full range of possible methods was available; here, despite the reduced range, a decision must be made. Thus the doctor must seek to fathom the secret of the patient's disease as quickly as possible, and not only the disease as an isolated phenomenon, but in context with the whole person. As soon as the patient begins to talk and describe his situation, it is necessary to weigh the volume of his words: what does it mean for this person to talk, to reveal himself? Initially, this is difficult. The words that are supposed to express the illness have an objective meaning. This meaning must be grasped as if by intuition, but everything subjective—the voice, the facial expressions, the brevity or length of the descriptions—is taken into account, perhaps indicating fear or fantasy or the need to make oneself important. And when he has to be undressed for an examination, it is once again important to maintain the right measure, exactly what is factually necessary.

In the hospital, the entire operation forms one unit through the cooperation of the doctors, nurses, and departments. Here you are alone: a doctor and a patient are together, and this is supposed to result in something that not only is objectively correct, but should also in the patient's mind create a kind of objective picture of his condition. In the hospital, the patient's statements are constantly being corrected; he may say what he wants—about himself, the doctors, the nurses—but the examinations speak an objective language. In the consulting room, these corrective moments largely disappear; the patient who goes home cannot be further pursued, but his statements can have considerable significance for the doctor's future.

The doctor must also not upset the patient unnecessarily—through words, the way in which he carries out the examinations, etc. and his actions must form a justifiable, coherent entity. And when he has done what he thinks is necessary and has arrived at a concrete diagnosis, provisional though it may be, he must formulate his instructions to the patient much more precisely than was necessary in the hospital. There, the doctor can make himself understood to the nurse in charge with half a word; he also knows to what extent she is reliable. If he orders a therapy, he knows that it will follow the prescribed course after he leaves, so that he only needs to supervise it from a distance. In the private practice consultation, on the other hand, the doctor gives his precise instructions to a person whom he most often does not know and cannot control; he does not know what the patient will make of them, how much he has understood of what has been said, which of them he decides to follow. So the doctor has to formulate the agenda much more clearly, even if he has no guarantee that it will be followed. Even if the patient comes to the consultation a second and third time and his condition has somehow changed for the better or for the worse, the doctor cannot be completely sure that this change is related to his instructions. Has the patient really taken his drops?

If it is something more serious, this uncertainty will be doubled: toward the patient on one side and toward the disease on the other, if the doctor cannot reconcile its course with his prescriptions. Various things are possible: there are cases where he can tell the patient outright that he did not follow the prescribed regimen; there are also those where the patient did not comply, but the doctor cannot tell: the patient can mislead the doctor by lying—and patients are particularly fond of lying—and thus jeopardize the entire treatment.

Soon the young doctor has a reckoning about all this; he has the feeling that he is largely at the mercy of others. In the hospital, a patient who refuses to comply can be discharged; the anonymity of the operation can easily tolerate this. A doctor, on the other hand, who has to build up his practice and make a name for himself, has to be considerate. He must not abandon a treatment at short notice, but must see how he can deal with a fruitless case. If he had to discharge a patient with an uncertain diagnosis, he would be left with a doubt, which can be very distressing, as there is often no way of remaining in contact with the patient. In the hospital, he could simply go and check again, if necessary reexamine the patient. But a town doctor calling a patient is a complete exception; he could easily be discredited as being over-anxious.

2. Dealing with Colleagues

Indirect Relationships

The doctor is in contact with all his colleagues: they are all representatives of conventional medicine. They generally reject anything that is not in line with it. By representing conventional medicine, they recognize certain basic truths that keep recurring in diagnosis as well as therapy. Everything builds on them: their personal style, their preferences, their intuition, their way of seeing the patient and his illness as an entity that is not unrelated to their own human entity. That the patient, incidentally, also wants to be seen as such an entity with its own particular character manifests itself in the fact that he, too, has his preferences in that he chooses this and not that doctor, even though both apply rather similar methods in their way of gauging the objective illness, and the true medical skill of the individual doctor is not apparent to the patient. For the patient cannot draw any conclusions about the efficiency of the doctor from the successes or failures of isolated cases known to him, as he lacks insight into the circumstances of the cases.

In contrast, the doctor has a greater ability to judge his colleagues; he is better informed about their skills.

However, he must not tier his dealings with them primarily according to his own assessment, but he should recognize and treat each one as a colleague from the outset. They have completed the same studies, possess the same willingness to help, and even if he does not always agree with a colleague on certain details, on questions of human empathy, he must nevertheless concede to him a rank equal to his own. Precisely because he himself knows how difficult it is to form an objective judgment of one's own performance, he will also be aware that he cannot judge the other person's modus operandi in its entirety. This lack of insight forces him to give his colleague the benefit of the doubt. He must assume that the other is doing the best he can.

If a patient comes to him who has experienced a failure with another doctor and is now being cured by himself, he will be wary of simply attributing the success to himself and his knowledge, as he does not know whether it was precisely what appeared to be a failure with the other doctor that created the preconditions for his own success. When he gets to hear what patients say about himself, his successes and failures, he will be amazed time and again at people's lack of judgment. (Many a patient complains about the doctor he left just because he didn't pay that doctor's bill. If one were to join in this rant, one would be helping to undermine the financial existence of one's colleague.) The doctor realizes how much his reputation is based on trivialities, but also how trivialities can jeopardize this reputation. Thus, he will distrust the patients' statements about a colleague and not discredit him.

Furthermore, if he were to agree with a patient's detrimental comments about a colleague, he would not only damage the reputation of the person concerned, but the reputation of all doctors practicing conventional medicine. He would also be encouraging presumptuous judgments by patients who do not know the true implications. That is why his statements about one of his colleagues should always be moderate and mediating. He does not have the full picture of his colleague's approach; the patient has even less. He knows how differently the same case can be approached, and with good reason.

So much for the indirect relationship with colleagues, as it is established by the patient.

The Direct Relationship

There are also cases in which the doctor must get in touch directly with the colleague whom the patient left. Not to shock him by telling him that the patient is now coming to him, but to inform himself about the course of the illness and the symptoms. It is then expected that, despite his irritation, the colleague will render a factual answer, since he himself expects to be informed just as correctly and openly in the reverse case. The individual doctor is so much a part of a team that he offers his colleague any help that will enable him to continue to manage the transferred case well.

If you temporarily take over patients from another doctor who is going on vacation or doing military service, you will naturally do nothing to bind such patients to you in such a way that they will not want to return to him upon his return. For them you are nothing but a substitute who should return them without any problem at the end of the substitution period. Some do not do this, under the pretext that some patients wished to stay with them. That is not collegial. They should at least remind the patients that they have placed their trust in the absent doctor and have only come to them by chance. Perhaps the patient can see the present doctor for another illness, but the treatment of the current illness should be completed with the doctor who initially treated it. By giving this advice, the substitute shows his own respect for his colleague. Anything that puts himself in a better and his colleague in a worse light is a breach of collegiality.

The treatment of a sick doctor creates a special situation. If you are dealing with someone who objectively has the same medical knowledge as you, but is subjectively biased by the fact that the illness is now his own, then you will largely respect his judgment. If he wants to be informed objectively, you are obliged to tell him everything you have realized. If he does not want this, you are equally obliged to remain silent, i.e., not to impose your own opinion on him, which evidently does not interest him. Although you will do what is necessary in your own opinion, you will not lecture him. If you are unclear about something, you are even more obliged to hold a consultation than you would be with a regular patient. It is not unusual for doctors to have abstruse illnesses or illnesses that take a different course than usual.

Doctors treat each other collegially, i.e., free of charge. In the past, it was customary to give a gift to a colleague at the end of a treatment; and as doctors were reluctant to give something useful for the practice, they usually resorted to atrocities. If you ask more precisely which doctors sick doctors choose for themselves, it turns out that it is almost always the professors. This puts a serious strain on their budget and time, but they still do not write any bills. In such cases, the colleague should definitely pay the appropriate fee. He can have his money delivered with a bouquet of flowers to emphasize the collegiality. But he should be aware that even a professor needs to be paid and has no use for a collection of impractical gifts. Nowadays the number of this type of gifts may have diminished, but the bad habit has not yet died out. And yet every doctor knows what a visit is worth. If the person treating him does not want to accept anything, he still has the option of transferring the fee to the doctors' fund, which supports doctors and widows of doctors.

There are cases in which the doctor comes to the conclusion that his patient should see a specialist. For example, he should see a surgeon to be operated on.

You have to ask him: "Whom would you like to see?" Often he may have no opinion of his own and asks back: "Whom would you advise me to see?" However, the doctor, and perhaps his family, may have long preferred a certain surgeon, even though this surgeon is not necessarily better than all the others. He will therefore not necessarily impose his own choice on his patient. If the patient is convinced of the quality of a specialist whom the doctor holds in lower esteem, then the doctor should not advise against it. This surgeon, too, has worked and holds his diploma. Incidentally, there can be a serious reason to advise the patient to see another doctor, but then the doctor should be able to justify this reason to anyone.

If he himself is ill or goes on vacation, he chooses a substitute at his discretion and lets his patients know. This does not force them to go to the designated substitute. It is enough when they know: this is my doctor's confidant.

In a city, every patient has often been to other doctors. If the doctor asks the patient about other physicians, he will do well not to trust the answer readily. He will much rather ask about previous illnesses, and thus come closer to the truth, and also realize how short the period of trust is for many patients. Very few people have a family doctor these days. The health insurance companies have thoroughly destroyed the system of general practice. Since the doctor costs practically nothing anymore (insurance pays, naturally), people have become accustomed to seeing the doctor as an official of the health insurance company. And when the doctor looks at his own patient base, he will realize that a certain percentage consists of loyal patients, but a larger percentage of passersby. They let themselves be treated, but regardless of the effort that one has put into them, the next time they go to someone else. They have no valid reasons for changing doctors. When a young doctor opens a practice, people will initially come to him for whom it is convenient at the time to have a doctor nearby, or those he knows from his student days or who have a vague relationship with his family. After a certain period of time, he is automatically included in the register of the health insurance companies. All members of the health insurance funds should actually receive the updated list of doctors annually. However, it can take five to seven years for a doctor to appear in the directory of all health insurance companies. When something is wrong with them, some people open their phone book, search under "throat doctors", for example, and then choose a doctor based on some external aspect: they have heard his name before, or the streetcar that leads to the office stops right in front of their house . . .

Proper collegiality would actually demand that every doctor have his fixed clientele. But because the system has collapsed, there are now a number of terms that are still intended to express collegiality but that have lost their relevance, ever more quickly in recent decades.

Patients are somewhat wary of collegiality. If they

have already been treated for a long time by one cardiologist, they feel somewhat guilty about confessing this to the new doctor when it is rather toward the previous one, whom they have left, that they should feel guilty. In the cities, where the health insurance system dominates everything, doctors have become accustomed to taking patients as they come, regardless of who has treated them before.

In rural areas, doctors rarely open a new practice, but usually take over an existing one when the old doctor retires. Then, of course, people come from the village and the area; the relationship is a different one. If the doctor is capable, and doesn't make any gross mistakes, people are proud of him and have no problem seeking his help. It is usually a bad sign when they start going to another village. The establishment of a new practice in the countryside almost always corresponds to a new need: for example, if a factory has opened in the village or the surrounding area, attracting workers, then the previously single practice may have to be shared, and a new doctor can establish himself alongside the one who is settled in. But this will rarely happen without fights, often bitter ones, if, for example, the population of the area is not dense enough. One may perish, the other may triumph. Rarely does the coexistence develop without rivalry. The normal scenario still is the taking over of an existing practice, which may be run by two doctors. The old doctor went from his larger village to the smaller one twice a week, and now a new doctor is starting his own practice in the latter, knowing from the outset that his prospects are limited.

3. Professional Secrecy

The Law

By law, a doctor may not discuss his patient's illness with anyone other than the patient himself or, in the case of minor children, with those responsible for them. But the system has long since been breached by the fact that the health insurance companies need to be informed of the diagnoses. This enables them to control the doctors. No one can, for instance, write down three visits in one day for a case of influenza. Actually, the diagnoses should only be known to the health insurance company's medical officer, but they are on the invoices so that all employees who have anything to do with them are aware of them as well, even in the case of a sexually transmitted disease, which is, of course, no longer tolerated in some places. The attitude of the patients also plays a role: some are indifferent to such disclosure, others are not. But precisely the tricky cases, such as venereal diseases, must be reported to the Department of Health; a patient who evades the regulations or infects others before being cured is taken care of until the risk of infection has passed. But suppose a maid in a family with an infant has gonorrhea—which puts the child at great risk, since he can go blind—and the mother calls to inquire, the doctor is not allowed to tell her about the maid's illness or even advise her to employ another one. If the person loses her job, she could sue him for it. Although professional secrecy is breached toward the health insurance companies and the authorities, it is not breached toward private individuals. All the doctor could do is to try and persuade the maid to give up her job on her own account. He must not force her to do so via the authorities, either, except in the case of public epidemics in which—as in a case of scarlet fever—the schools are closed.

Among doctors, who are both bound by professional secrecy, talking about a patient is permitted. It is part of collegiality to inform each other. Where there is a need, it is customary; where there is none, it is tolerated. Naturally, a patient can release the doctor from professional secrecy for his case. He must, in fact, do so if he has made a corresponding commitment toward a health insurance company. Or if he wants to take out a life insurance policy and comes for an examination. If the doctor finds an illness that will shorten his life, he is obliged to inform the insurance company, since the patient has agreed in writing that the findings will be disclosed to the insurance company.

If the patient is an adult, the doctor may not disclose anything to family members, unless the patient has instructed him to do so. When talking to family members, it is not about medical insights, but about prognoses that are important for the patient's environment. For example, how long an illness will last, in case the relatives already know or suspect the essentials.

However, the patient always has the right to object to such disclosures. A meeting should only take place if there is a danger to life in the home, and even then not with the entire family, but with those responsible. Nurses who need to be aware are also bound by professional secrecy; they too are not allowed to talk to relatives, even though they often do—against their better judgment.

I–He, I–You

Two things make up the medical profession. One is the science that deals with the disease and knows the ways to cure it. Then there is the sick person who comes to the doctor with his human need and expects a certain form of humanity from him.

There is the borderline case in which the second factor seems to have been eliminated. A surgeon may see the patient—who has already been put to sleep—for the first time when he is brought into the operating theater; another surgeon has made the diagnosis, on the basis of which he knows what he will have to do. Or a seriously injured patient is brought in who has to be operated on immediately, regardless of how the patient is feeling in other respects; without the operation he would surely die.

But this is not the norm. In most cases, a patient comes to the doctor and reports his illness himself; the doctor has to go through the patient's subjective statements to arrive at an objective diagnosis. And that is not the only thing he has to do. He has to treat the patient, who has entrusted him with something from his life, as this unique person who perhaps expects more from him than the quick repair of an isolated damage, namely, somehow the healing of everything that is not well in him: his overall physical weakness that predisposes him to his particular illness and has led him to attempt suicide, or this lack of energy that prevents him from leading a sensible life-style, or his personal problems that cause him sleepless nights.

The doctor's first relationship with the patient is that of I-and-He, the second, that of I-and-You.

In order to arrive at this "You", the doctor cannot rely solely on the patient's statements. He must mobilize elements of his own ego and prepare a home for the other person with himself. He must take the time to deal with the problems of the other person who has surrendered himself to him. He must undertake a contemplation of the "You", and this within his own concept of life. If the patient has a right to the doctor's personality, the doctor has a duty to take his patient as personally as he is. The mutual relationship that develops on a personal level initiates a process for the doctor that requires him to come to terms with himself, because only then can he himself reach maturity. This process requires stillness and silence; it appeals to the doctor's duty of confidentiality.

This duty does not consist only in the negative, i.e., that no statements may be made. It is also something positive: the doctor must remain silent in order to gain the necessary insight. Nor is it mere discretion, unless one were to give this term its spiritual sense of *discretio spiritualis* and then understand it as an essential factor of the doctor's human involvement with the patient. In this profound sense, the required medical confidentiality is the core, albeit not the origin, of medical contemplation; out of it grows the doctor's actual personal nature, that which distinguishes him from other doctors in his profession and mission, that which constitutes his unique personality. In his inner attentive listening, in his contemplative vision, lies the opposite of a relation to himself, namely, that relation to the "You", which as such determines the doctor's actual growing into the "I". Confidentiality is not the duty to forget, but to keep something within oneself that adheres more firmly and concretely because it must not be externalized. Precisely because it must be kept secret, it occupies us more deeply. Because we are used to passing everything on so easily, it is not really assimilated; but the real presents itself again and again under unexpected aspects and should thus become the preferred object of inner contemplation.

The doctor's professional action is largely conditioned by technology, science, learned measures. His contemplation arises from his contact with the patient. From both technical knowledge and the insight resulting from contemplation, however, a *second action* arises. It is a refined action because it has passed through the doctor's personality. It is the fruit not only of his experience with this type of illness, but of his experience with this person in this illness. Through this medical contemplation, the patient regains his primary dignity.

Stimulating Literature

The people with whom the doctor deals and who demand help from him very often offer him only fleeting, impressionistic snapshots. Suffering and questions that revolve around suffering create the foreground; but a background that would provide consistency and interpretability for everything is missing. In order to be able to help, the doctor needs to complete the images presented to him. He cannot be satisfied with getting to know people merely in the small sections of their lives as presented during consultation hours, even if the encounters are numerous. Nor can he be satisfied with supplementing the missing information with medical and paramedical literature, for instance, psychiatric literature, and to study the people in these books that are specifically tailored toward the doctor. There he will always find them reduced, labeled as a case of illness. In order to be able really to live with sick people, in order to understand their everyday existence through the excerpt that is shown more explicitly to him as a doctor, he also needs a number of images that have nothing to do with the particular medical field, that rest, as it were, in themselves, images such as those born of the imagination of a poet or novelist, perhaps also the simple descriptions of someone who knows how to tell stories and describe his fellow human beings, without particular finesse, but out of human proximity. What matters is that the barriers of the doctor's way of looking at things fall away and that the reading doctor takes in figures that possess the fullness of human totality.

Perhaps it is the image of a person who is in the same room with others, who wants to do the same thing that everyone else does as a matter of course, and an incomprehensible power, the power of illness, prevents him from doing so. Or the image of a man in a factory yard; all the others do their work easily, only he can no longer do it, and the task weighs down on him like a hundredweight until he collapses. A thousand situations are possible, all of which lie outside the narrow confines of consultation hours, sickrooms, and hospitals and yet present as much of a reality for the suffering. After all, the patient is not a chimera composed of lots of pathological symptoms. He is a human being among human beings who can only be understood in the unbroken context of life. Detached from all the habits of school, science, and diagnostics, the doctor must learn first to see this person in his true, unique humanity.

He must see as Rilke saw the epileptic walking down the Boulevard St-Michel, discovering him with the almost incomprehensible acuteness of an eye that is not medical but poetic, describing him at first with a kind of cool objectivity, then becoming more and more moved by what he sees, until he reacts to it as a poet, with his whole being, and finally can no longer help but walk behind the sick man and keep him in his sight. He must have a kind of inner readiness to grasp, to hold, to follow, to help—not as a doctor, but as someone who simply knows and understands. It is also by no means merely the pleasure of poetic creation that has entangled Rilke into this adventure, a form of pleasure that can be found in the creative overcoming of suffering, too, but pure humanity that addresses and retroactively shapes our humanity. He narrates the course of the crisis in such a way that the illness takes on something sublime. The illness that renders the man helpless and robs him of the possibility of expression does not hide itself. It is there, obvious, on the street; it offers itself to the poet free of charge; it makes itself available to him in order to help him create his work, so that the poet's compassion is not even the primary phenomenon, but a response to the prior revelation of the illness. The poet gives in creating; but his gift is based on the preceding gift of the patient's selfless showing of himself. The sick person is a victim whose sacrifice comes to fruition in the poet.

But the doctor's literary occupation is by no means only about the sick. It is about the human encounter in general. It is about the expansion of one's own narrow focus into the general human perspective. This expansion is at the same time the true relaxation from the tenseness of one's own constriction of the mind. Reading many and different kinds of things can be the best form of relaxation. One encounters a wealth of characters none of whom want anything from you, who live their own lives, but whose existence is open to the reader, a gift for anyone who deals with people. This abundance enlivens in us what is in danger of becoming monotonous because of our profession. And the more colorful and diverse the image of man that the doctor takes in, the more capable he will be of differentiating his diagnosis and treatment in cases of seemingly identical problems, distracting patients from a perhaps biased image of themselves, and leading them to a deeper truth. And again, not on the basis of abstract and general theories about the human soul, as modern psychology offers them to the doctor, but with the help of direct, concrete knowledge of the person himself. Not artificially interpreting on the basis of preconceived schemes, but naturally reading from the living image of the real, present person.

This requires more than just a description of the individual in his isolation. It requires the milieu, nature, the home and the foreign, the great backdrops of the landscape even in their seeming indifference to man: stones, forest, clouds and sky . . . and man in the middle of it all, acting, suffering, making decisions, a moving point in a still life whom we follow and observe, but who is not concerned with us observers. He, uninvolved, before us who are involved, who for once do not need to see him with our eyes, but who can look through his eyes, at the landscape, the village, fate. Sometimes this moving point may not be there at all: the poetry leads us deep into pristine nature—and man is represented in it in nothing but the eloquent artistic expression of the poet himself. This is where we gain complete distance; we rest from people, in a kind of Sabbath that gives us the strength to face a new week among them. With that we have arrived at an edge, an edge, however, that is no less essential to the picture than the center. An edge at which, instead of the book, there may just as well be the symphony, sculpture, painting, or architecture. Every kind of art will stimulate the doctor; and his response to every work of art will be a new service, because the artist himself has produced it to serve: so that what he feels called to may become reality. Not at all, if he really is an artist, with any thought of benefit and making himself useful, but simply for the sake of the radiant power of beauty. But what is true of the work of art is no less true of every real encounter with a person facing you: the unintentional nature of it possesses a fecundity that is like gratitude for the selflessness of the pure encounter.

III

HEALTHY AND SICK

1. The Problem of Health

Illness is the disturbance of a state that is called health. This can be described as the natural and expected course of bodily functions: such as sleeping and waking, eating, digestion, bowel movement, etc. If they function "normally", the person does not even take notice of them. He only becomes aware of their significance when they begin to malfunction or fail completely. In this way, one would describe health in just a few words and rather list in negative terms the things that are contrary to it. One would then arrive at the one definition of health by subtraction.

In concrete terms, however, it would remain difficult to determine this state of being healthy, since everyone has some weaknesses and deficiencies. Such deficiencies, however, are so familiar to the individual that as long as the general functioning of the body continues and he is not prevented from working, he does not feel compelled to take any decisive action and therefore does not describe himself as ill.

If, however, an adult dies by some accident and an autopsy is conducted, one will usually notice various signs of more or less pronounced diseases, which, according to his own statements—perhaps shortly before his death—did not trouble him in the least. Perhaps the illness was so slight or so latent that it had not yet become noticeable through any outward symptoms, or the deceased had resigned himself to the symptoms, incorporated them into his life-style in such a way that they did not significantly interfere with his work, his enjoyment of life, his habits. Perhaps, even if the symptoms had become more severe, he would not have gone to the doctor because of them. Perhaps something far more minor, but something that caused him pain, that became a hindrance, would have brought him to the doctor.

Therefore, neither the subjective severity of symptoms nor the patient's complaints and the impairment of his work are sufficient to judge an illness in terms of its severity, duration, and prognosis. What really takes place on the inside and can endanger life and what disturbs the patient on the outside need not be in any evident relation to each other. A woman with breast cancer may be unaware of her illness for a long time: she feels no fatigue or disinclination to work; her sleep, appetite, and general mood are undisturbed, and by the time an external circumstance, a chance touch or perception of the tumor draws her attention to it, she is already condemned to death, with only a short period of agonizing suffering ahead of her. Another woman of the same age may have a glandular disease of the breast that torments her, causes her sleepless nights, and disfigures her: she rushes to the doctor, who, despite the severe symptoms, declares her mildly ill; her tumor will have no effect on her life-span or ability to work.

If a patient comes to the consultation to find out whether he is healthy, the doctor will first examine him briefly, carry out some functional tests, perhaps look for some signs of illness that are common at his age, and then dismiss him with the assurance that there is nothing wrong with him. And perhaps this is only because an examination, which he did not carry out, would have revealed the presence of a disease that would require surgery.

Thus, "health" can only be determined imprecisely. Below the surface, there may be things that are either impossible to diagnose or require a more sophisticated method. If someone wants to know at all costs whether he is healthy, it will not be possible to assure him of this with absolute certainty; one can only check at regular intervals what is medically testable. Such a person would spend most of his life at the doctor's, and the preoccupation with his health would become the focus of his attention. Since this is unreasonable, and since there would also never be enough doctors to carry out such general examinations, one should be content to judge one's health by the fact that one can continue to work as usual and that there are no significant deficits.

Therefore a strong dose of trust is needed: first in nature, in our own body, but then also in God. We trust that what cannot be verified corresponds approximately to what can be verified. We can recognize the quality of our sleep in the fact that we are rested in the morning. Certain glands with internal secretion elude examination. But if everything appears to be in balance, there is no point in worrying, in artificially suspecting antagonisms within ourselves. Such basic trust is undoubtedly also most conducive to the preservation of health.

And because we know that trust is necessary in matters of health, we also trust our doctor, to whom we entrust the judgment about our health and illness and its potential severity. A patient must know from the outset that he cannot judge subjectively conspicuous symptoms of illness in terms of their objective severity. Their conspicuousness has led him to suspect a certain illness and to consult the doctor, but very often the latter will be able to cure the patient, who considers himself seriously ill, by simple means, whereas in the case of someone who thinks it almost superfluous to go to the doctor, the latter may have to present him with the prospect of an operation, a long treatment that perhaps promises little success.

The Doctor's Behavior

The sick person who comes to the doctor because he is suffering from irritating symptoms is unable to see through the objective correlations. He experiences them separately. Often he only becomes really ill during the consultation, at the moment when he learns the name of the illness, i.e., when he no longer merely feels individual symptoms, but sees himself belonging to a category of illness. It is not unusual for the doctor to see this categorization becoming a crucial experience for the patient. The patient may know of a similar case in his family and so on, and spontaneously makes suggestions for a treatment that is familiar to him from other cases.

At the moment when the name of the disease is pronounced, the doctor can engage most deeply in the patient's life. The shock that occurs when that name is mentioned opens up something in the patient that the doctor can tap into. He is no longer an outsider as before; a new relationship has been established between him and the patient. The doctor will immediately try to provide the patient with the right attitude toward his illness. If it is severe, he will say a word about the meaning of the suffering in a way that is comprehensible to the patient and helps him to adjust to it. Furthermore, the patient, even if he does not understand everything, should accept the measures taken by the doctor and required by the seriousness of the situation, and in such a way that he does not just passively comply with the instructions, but also personally trusts the doctor, which excludes any desire to know better and any equal say. All this does not need to be explained at length, it will express itself in the doctor's overall attitude.

In a milder case, the doctor will show the patient the way out of the illness, point out to him the success that awaits him if he complies with the instructions.

Where no success is to be expected, the doctor must gradually break this to the patient, even if not at the first visit. This way, in the heavy times that will follow, the patient will not find any contradictions to what the doctor predicted, and indeed will have stronger confidence in him because of the correct diagnosis. If he wants to remain objective, in this situation there is only one choice for the doctor when facing the patient: full discretion. He must not identify himself with the illness in such a way that illness and doctor merge into a single concept for the patient; but under no circumstances must he leave the patient now. The patient must have the certainty that the doctor accompanies him in his illness, empathizes with what he feels, and that this human closeness will help him to bear the illness properly. However, the doctor has no right to exaggerate his role in any way, to play up the illness and its consequences in such a way that in case of a healing he looks like a magician.

The first step is to introduce the patient to the new state of being ill without turning it into something definitive, whatever the prognosis may be.

If the illness is mild and curable, the doctor must help the patient not to see the illness tragically, to retain the prospect of recovery, also not to flee from being ill, to accept it now as something decisive. He should not see it as a mere accident that will disappear tomorrow, but rather should experience the state of being ill at least somewhat consciously. Although he should under no circumstances become a hypochondriac, he must not reject what providence suggests to him with this illness. If the doctor knows anything of these correlations, i.e., if he does not see illness as something purely determined by fate, then he will be aware of his responsibility and disclose to the patient as much of it as he is able to grasp.

If the illness is fatal, this responsibility deepens even more: the approaching death becomes a more immediate part of it. A demand arises that grows beyond the mere illness. Some of this the patient must hear. If the illness is a chronic one that will probably last for a long time without major changes, there can be no question of settling in the state of illness; this would inevitably turn the patient into an egoist: with his illness he would become the center of attention for himself and his surroundings; the sense for the everyday life of healthy people around him and also for the promised life hereafter would be lost.

At the moment when the doctor tells the patient his diagnosis, he must give a brief overview of the nature and course of the illness so that the patient at least knows what the near future will probably look like. At this point, the doctor can already give him a few instructions that can help him to turn the period of illness into a productive time. And if in this situation he touches on the patient's intimate world, he should do so not only as a medical professional, but as a person with his own worldview. Of course, the patient should never for a moment have the feeling that an alien worldview is being imposed on him, to some extent because he is in the defenseless state of being ill. On the other hand, the patient must also be aware that the doctor is not a mere machine by whose operation his health will be restored, but is a person who, even if he has limited skills, is nevertheless a personality with his own worldview. The patient cannot demand that the doctor should abandon the wholeness of his person so as to attend to him only as a technician. Even if the doctor does not involve him in his private life, he still takes him into the sphere of his responsible consideration; for if he is there to help the patient—and that is what the patient demands—he cannot do so in a completely uninvolved manner. It is in the patient's interest that the doctor does not merely adhere to the few symptoms that are presented to him, but sees him, the patient, as a whole person, whom he certainly must treat as a whole person. Based on this relationship, the doctor also knows that his patient has not waited until the consultation to think about illness, life, and death. But for the patient, the abstract thoughts now become concrete: he enters a new phase of life, and since he is now dependent on the doctor, he remains exposed to his influence. It is precisely this exposure that requires the doctor to exercise the aforementioned full discretion and fair play.

In most cases, the patient does not realize how sensitive and vulnerable he is right now. He is shaken because he has to adjust to a new state of life. He went to the doctor voluntarily, now he has to yield: first to the illness, but also to the doctor, who will not be able to carry out his treatment without employing his own subjectivity. Everything that previously made up the solid framework of the patient's existence, everything with which he has furnished it, begins to falter, as the more or less thought-out principles he has set himself are for the most part not sustainable in the face of the new condition. Naturally, his worldview largely corresponded to that of a healthy person, and, unreflectingly, he considered this worldview unchangeable. Certainly, the child's worldview had given way to the adult's, the apprentice's to the master's, that is to say, the disposer's; but only in the rarest of cases did he realize that he had become a slave to the image he had envisaged and that his freedom within this image was quite limited, so that now that the old image no longer holds up, he cannot simply dispose of this freedom anew, but must subordinate everything altogether to the demands of his illness. It is enough that he is now confined to bed for five weeks, will suffer pain, will have to have an operation, and thus what he demands and expects from his existence takes on a completely different character: what he naively took for granted so far is supplanted by the situation now imposed on him. Things, on the other hand, that he hardly suspected, hardly wanted to acknowledge, become concrete and prioritized; he no longer understands how he could have passed them by so indifferently. What he is now experiencing is unique, forceful, and decisive; it appears to him as an unknown entity that he absolutely must deal with. The doctor is well aware of this situation; he experiences it almost daily. He is therefore inclined from the outset to offer the patient a helping hand, to show him that his present experience is just as true and meaningful as all the previous things that are now fading.

From this ever-recurring experience ultimately emerges that which constitutes the doctor's professional ethos. He cannot pass by the experience that his patient goes through as if it were something accidental that is simply part of the job. If he has a sense of professional responsibility, he understands that he must personally participate in this experience, that this shock to his neighbor's existence must resonate in him and challenge him at the very core of his professional work. If he did not deepen the commonality of experience of patient and doctor for himself as well, if he regarded the patient's illness only as an external phenomenon from which the suffering person remained excluded, his technical and scientific skills would perhaps not suffer, but the human in him would increasingly atrophy. In the end, he would only see the disease, no longer the sick person who suffers it, or see the sick person only as a necessary evil. He would prefer to have the disease in front of him in its purest form; the person would then only be the cause of its occurrence—just as bacilli are observed under the microscope and not the tissue in which they are found. In doing so, he would strip his field of action of the human element, on both sides, in fact, the patient's as well as his own, and demonstrate that he can only be partially considered a doctor: as long as symptoms are pathologically interpretable and, scientifically speaking, an effective therapy is available for them. Basically, he would not be practicing a vocation at all—no one would have called him: neither God nor the suffering human being—but merely practicing a craft that requires a limited amount of artistry from him, a skill limited to technique. It is inevitable, then, that the patient becomes more and more deeply disappointed by this impoverishment. He experiences how the illness transforms his inner life, but at the same time he realizes that the doctor remains outside this process of transformation. In fact, the patient would ultimately have to take on a doctor's role toward the doctor by revealing his human inadequacy to him and showing him that mere science is not sufficient to grasp his case.

The doctor thus recognizes the extent to which he is in a mutual relationship with his patient, even if due to his knowledge he is the superior in it. Both of them are involved in a larger context that forces them to deal with the ultimate questions of existence. If the doctor is not already a person of faith but possesses a sense of responsibility, and through his solidarity with the patient sees himself confronted with the essential question of meaning, he cannot evade the final big question of "Why" and can ultimately only search for the "Because" beyond the human relationship. If in his patient's state of subjection, and perhaps also through his own efforts, he experiences something that can no longer be adequately grasped in purely human terms, he will be forced to transfer the solution to the riddles to the source of things. And because his relationship to the patient points him there, he also senses that the vitality of this relationship cannot simply break off with the patient's last breath, or with the fact that he has educated the patient to bear the thought of death and to die manfully, but that the bond that has been formed lasts beyond that. Certainly there are also atheistic doctors for whom death is the end of everything; somewhere they have deliberately marked a point beyond which they do not want to ask any further. They have resolved to stop.

2. *The Problem of Truth*

Its Aspects

We arrive at a similar result when we ask the question of what can be described as truth in the medical process. The doctor has the advantage of having objective knowledge about illnesses and healing processes that the patient does not have. But this objective knowledge has its limits and is not immutable. The patient, for his part, has the advantage that he feels his illness, experiences it in a manner that corresponds to the mutability of life, and that can approximate the objective medical insights or also distance itself from them. The question is how these two forms of truth relate to each other, whether they can be brought to congruence at all.

To begin with, the patient knows that the doctor possesses trustworthy knowledge that was tested by science and that he acquired himself. An injection is needed here, an operation there, and so on. This knowledge is clearly superior to that of the patient, which is why the patient submits to it without further ado. Thanks to his objective knowledge, the doctor is able to help a fellow human being. But his knowledge is not an absolute one; after all, medical science is in a constant state of development, things it considers correct today will be abandoned tomorrow. Surrounding the core of medicine are sciences such as physics, mechanics, botany, and zoology, each of which in turn goes its own way and the new achievements of which also benefit and change medicine. These advances are not straightforward; they occur in jolts. And the effects of each of these sciences—chemistry, for instance—on medicine must first be tested by the latter. New remedies are advertised and enthusiastically adopted by many doctors, which after a few years prove to be harmful in a certain respect and have to be withdrawn from the market. Thus the doctor will realize the relativity of the truth that applies to him and remain critical toward it, even though he does not need to tell the patient anything—at least anything that does not concern the patient—about the questionable aspects he is aware of. Above all, he must bear in mind that not all people react in the same way to the same remedies or precautions, because when it comes to his life system, each person has his own truth. My flu is not your flu; what helps me may have no effect on you.

This turns our attention back to what—with a certain degree of caution—we call the patient's truth, which can exhibit very different layers. The sick person is first and foremost a human being with his own fate, not a mere case. This does not mean that he is unique, for he is largely subject to the laws that the doctor knows and assumes to be valid for the physical nature of every human being. That is also why the sick person submits to the medical artistry and cannot demand that every decision of the doctor be explained and justified to him. With his limited knowledge, he very soon reaches the point where he must entrust himself to the knowledge and responsibility of the doctor. Again and again, it turns out that the proper examinations carried out by the doctor on the patient reveal something different from what the patient meant, felt in terms of symptoms, and believed to be objectively true.

The discrepancy between subjective and objective truth can become extreme in patients. Almost forty years ago, I met a young nurse in Leysin, in a kind of preventorium where no seriously ill patients, only those in need of convalescence or people with closed tuberculosis were staying; if they were diagnosed with open, i.e., infectious TB, they were discharged immediately. This girl, Solange, called Soso, had just been diagnosed with open TB; she had to move to a sanatorium. She was in shock and began to describe her future—not cynically, but with a kind of inexorability: "I know exactly what will happen next. I will go to the sanatorium, and after a few months I will be told: 'The illness appears to be more serious than we thought, but it is by no means hopeless. You will now be taken to Lausanne because the climatic conditions will be better for you there.' There I will lie in a room with twelve others. And at some point they will say: 'We want to move you to a small room so that you can get more rest; they will also be able to give you better food there, which is not available in the big room.' And one day they will push me into the corridor, and then it will soon be over. But I have enough insight into my condition not to believe a word of what they tell me." There was something frightening about the sick woman's clairvoyance of what was to come. She knew in advance how little she could trust the "truth" that would be offered to her. She also knew how she wanted to defend herself in advance against being lied to like this. I saw Solange two more times, the second time in the small room in Lausanne. She: "Now I'm in the small room because they can give me wine here. . . . As soon as I feel better, I'll get back to the big room, and from there I'll go back to Leysin at last for after-treatment." She spoke in a small, coughing voice that was barely audible. Suddenly she looked at me and said: "You believe what I'm saying, don't you?" And I said: "Yes."

This story has always haunted me; it would probably haunt any doctor. The subjectively recognized truth initially prevailed over the "objective" truth—which the patient recognized as untruth—until she had distanced herself so much from her initial realization that a clarification about the truth no longer seemed possible, or at least no longer feasible.

This extreme case exemplifies many similar illnesses where people are driven into a nervous disorder by some kind of excessive demand that narrows their worldview and places them at the center of everything. Everything that concerns the sick person becomes excessively important; anything that concerns others is of little or no importance to him. It cannot be said that he is a liar, but he has constructed a purely personal truth for himself and walled himself into it. In the event that the person in question is also physically ill, the doctor is faced with a difficult question: Will medical knowledge be enough to cure him or must another level of truth be activated here: that of personal existence? Should he not reveal to the patient his personal worldview, or at least something of it, in addition to all the factual care? Give him something of a deeper truth that must occupy him, which he encounters like an obstacle, until he finally realizes that the obstacle lies, not in what is being communicated, but in himself?

We are less concerned here with the likewise important point that psychopathology, too, has its history and development, which the therapist has to deal with on his part, but would rather refer beyond this level to the last level, the one that ultimately matters. The meaning of the whole, which transcends every human being, lies in the Absolute, in God. Ultimately, only the view of the absolute can break open the relativities and imminent absolutizations of merely "objective" and merely "subjective" truth and also open them up to each other in a fruitful way. When the Absolute, God, opens Himself up to people, as in Christianity, then God is not just a mystery—He will always be that—but something in which the believer can also participate. If God reveals Himself as love for us, then we live within this love through our openness to our fellow men and our devotion to them, which is then no longer merely sociological or ethical, but has the depth and intensity of the religious. What we now implement as love is greater than what we can grasp, because its source lies in God. Here and here alone the doctor's knowledge and skill and the patient's personal knowledge and experience can encounter each other in a valid way.

Hospitals run by Christian nurses, often women

religious, show how the most favorable atmosphere for medical work can be drawn out of the highest Christian truth. Out of the truth of revelation the Sisters live the actuality of charity in their daily lives. Naturally, they must try to keep pace with medical science in their training, but they must integrate it into something more comprehensive. And the doctor working in their midst cannot remain indifferent to this atmosphere. Of course, doctors should be good professionals—and not preach Christianity instead—but professionals within a space of comprehensive truth, who know that they are taken into responsibility by it and are thus able to measure up to what the sick person as such demands of them.

Every truth is somehow participation, but participation in God is the highest truth. Recognizing it in faith means participating in it. And from the point of view of this truth, the doctor's responsibility becomes participation in his neighbor, the sick person; it is the illness that imparts this special encounter of I and You. The proper development in the life of a doctor goes in this direction: that in him the sense for the living becomes ever more alive in the taking on and accompanying of the patient, whether his future is healing or death.

Impressions from Consultation Hours

Klara. One Pentecost Saturday evening, probably in 1932, I was called to see some complete strangers, whose doctor was away for Sunday or a few days. There were twin children lying in two beds. The mother told me in the hallway that one of them had had a severe case of pneumonia and was better now, but she was still worried and asked if I would please have a look at the child. When I entered the room I went to one of the beds. No, no, that was the healthy child, the sick one was lying there! I examine the child, the pneumonia was over, everything was fine so far, Klara could be allowed to get up, but Anna in the other bed gives me the impression of a sick child. The mother doesn't want to hear about it. May I examine her? No! The next morning a phone call: come immediately, Anna is dying. When I got there, she was dead. Pneumonia, much more severe than her sister's. For the mother, the seriously ill child had still been healthy on Saturday; she was so absorbed by Klara's illness that she no longer had an eye for Anna.—We are not provided with a medical mandate that would allow us to visit every sick person, but only those entrusted to us. Actually, it was already too much that I had insisted on being allowed to examine the other child. From a medical ethical point of view, it was wrong.

Kaspar was a touching little man who regularly brought me his wife's urine in a small bottle; she was diabetic. I saw her every week, and in between I examined the urine that Kaspar brought. He was very much henpecked, the woman was bossy. Her diabetes was an easy matter. You simply had to prove to her again and again that she had eaten too many pastries and advise her to switch to other foods that she loved less. But the entire household trembled before this illness! One day, the urine Kaspar brought me contained about 7% sugar instead of the usual 0.5% or 0.25%. I said to him: "For God's sake, what has your wife been eating? I don't understand this, even if she has eaten a lot of sweets . . ." Kaspar smiled a little bashfully and confessed that this time it was his urine in the bottle. He had been feeling tired for a long time and kept having dizzy spells. He had long suspected something like this, but when he spoke to his wife about it, she laughed at him and wouldn't tolerate this kind of competition in the house. He died three weeks later from his diabetes, while his wife is still alive today.

Emma was a maid whom I had to treat for years for all sorts of ailments that never quite made sense to me. I often talked to her about that. I didn't quite trust the situation, but there wasn't much I could do. She kept coming back for doctor's notes: so that she wouldn't have to wax the floors at her job because her kidneys were too weak to do so. Or for an increase in her sugar ration because her stomach needed sugar. Or she asked for a note stating that her heart was not strong enough to take part in the air-raid drills. One fine day she was back at the consultation. "So, Emma, what kind of note do you want today?" She: "A note that I'm completely healthy." "What's happened?" "I'm just getting married. And he doesn't want a sick wife." That was the first note I gave her with a clear conscience. Since then she has disappeared, so that one can assume that she is healthy by virtue of the note.

Ida was a sales clerk in a supermarket. She came in with severe sciatica. Sciatica is one of the few conditions where you are largely dependent on the patient's testimony. If a patient knows what symptoms sciatica causes, he can tell the doctor what he wants; the doctor has no means of proving that he does not have the condition. So Ida, a lively girl, came with sciatica and at the same time with the wish to be treated in the hospital. I admitted her to the hospital. Soon afterward she developed quite a high fever, which clouded the picture of sciatica. At first I didn't know what she might have. Eventually I took her into the bathroom and asked her what was really wrong with her life, why she was simulating this fever like the sciatica? She immediately confessed that she wanted to enter a convent and had no way of persuading her parents to let her go. So she thought that if she were really ill, her parents would take pity on her and think: better a daughter in a convent than one in the grave. I was rather taken aback by these premises for a religious life. But she entered a convent three weeks later, and I was present at her profession. She became a good Sister.

Katharina is the saint of her parish, who sacrifices herself endlessly for a healthy woman, and in the end it is she who dies. She is seventy years old, has been unable to work for several years, and is supported by the state: It was terrible, she said, that she was a burden to the community. The state paid for her health insurance, so she rarely had herself examined so as not to harm the state. When a neighbor named B., who lived in the same house, developed rheumatic symptoms and could only move with difficulty, Katharina became a slave to B. No effort was too great for her; she did everything, really everything, that she could do for the other woman. Every time B. had the slightest problem, Katharina had to tell me to come immediately. Finally, one Friday evening, I was called back to the apartment and told that this time it was for Katharina. She was lying very stiffly on a narrow sofa that had served as her bed for more than three years, as B. didn't allow her to sleep in her own room, where there was a proper bed, but always wanted to have her at hand at night. Katharina had agreed to this because she felt healthy enough to be allowed to help a sick person. When I had examined her and had to tell her that she was seriously ill and absolutely had to go to hospital, her first reply was: No, she couldn't do that, B. didn't like being alone. I went back the next morning because a neighbor had called me: Katharina was unconscious and dying. The moment I entered, she opened her eyes and when I asked her what had happened, she said: "Not much, I'm sure, but I think B. is worried, comfort her!" Then she was indeed taken to hospital and died the following night. When I saw B. again on Monday, she said: "Yes, yes, Katharina really spoiled me so that now I can't move at all!'' That was the entire eulogy.

Mrs. Meyer. In the very early days of my practice, a woman came in from the waiting room with a very big belly. She could barely hold herself upright. She told me that she had been suffering from incredible back pain since yesterday and that it was radiating toward her stomach. Me: ''In your condition, that's not surprising.'' She: ''In my condition?'' ''Yes, at the end of the pregnancy!'' ''But I'm not pregnant.'' Me to myself: If only I had kept quiet! I examined her: they were barely able to get her to the hospital by cab, and half an hour later the baby was there. But before that I confirmed with her: she had had six children and was sure that the seventh was on the way. In the third month then, she had been to a doctor who told her she wasn't pregnant, in the fourth month she was there again: she felt movements, the doctor laughed at her. And so she spent the last few months in the certainty of not being pregnant.

Sister Margarita was examined by a doctor many years ago, who told her that she had cardiac insufficiency as a result of the illness she had just overcome. ''You must take it easy and stay on a diet.'' He gave her precise instructions on how she should behave. She obediently followed his instructions, it didn't even occur to her that they could be temporary, that this diagnosis involving the heart was only relevant for a certain period of time, and that the symptoms were therefore reversible. When I examined her many years later and she told me that she was suffering from heart disease, I couldn't find anything at all. She was, however, not exaggerating her symptoms, for since she had consistently been on a specific lean diet and meticulously measured all her movements and exertions, over time her physical fitness had diminished. This was a tough call: it was not possible suddenly to deny her illness, because she could not from one day to the next live the life of a healthy person. And all that had happened must also not be represented as meaningless. On the other hand, one could not leave everything as it was. . . . Her case, like the previous one, clearly shows how sometimes too much weight can be put on the doctor's word.

A young nun has hemorrhoids. One would never have thought of this; from the description she gave of the illness, one would have thought she was suffering from a severe illness of the lower part of the intestine. She described everything to me so drastically and gravely that I got the impression her entire life had been affected by this illness and that her main spiritual achievement lay in the bearing of this suffering. When I finally examined her, I found a small harmless hemorrhoid, which disappeared within a few days under the most common treatment. It was certainly not that she wanted to exaggerate her symptoms, but she, and perhaps above all those around her, lacked insight into the scale of things: the comparison with other illnesses. This hemorrhoid was taken as an absolute suffering, and within this absoluteness the Sister's symptoms seemed so essential that a large part of her strength was taken up in perceiving and experiencing them properly. And because everyone else thought she had a serious illness, they would have certainly considered themselves guilty if they had taken the matter a little more lightly.

IV

THE CHRISTIAN DOCTOR

Scripture

Chapter 38 of the Book of Sirach talks about the physician:[1]

> Honor the physician with the honor due him,
>   according to your need of him,
>   for the Lord created him;
> for healing comes from the Most High,
>   and he will receive a gift from the king.
> The skill of the physician lifts up his head,
>   and in the presence of great men he is admired.
> The Lord created medicines from the earth,
>   and a sensible man will not despise them.
> . . . .
> And he gave skill to men
>   that he might be glorified in his marvelous works.
> By them he heals and takes away pain;
>   the pharmacist makes of them a compound.
> His works will never be finished;
>   and from him health is upon the face of the earth.
> My son, when you are sick do not be negligent,
>   but pray to the Lord, and he will heal you.

[1] For Scripture quotes, I have based my translation on that of the Revised Standard Version, Second Catholic Edition.—Trans.

Give up your faults and direct your hands aright,
and cleanse your heart from all sin.
. . . .
And give the physician his place, for the Lord created him;
let him not leave you, for there is need of him.
There is a time when success lies in the hands of physicians,
for they too will pray to the Lord
that he should grant them success in diagnosis
and in healing, for the sake of preserving life.

An astounding passage that describes in brief strokes the entire complexity of the relation between the natural and the religious realm, between an immediate relationship and one that is mediated by doctor and medicine. There is a relationship between the patient and God that is to be mediated through his trust in the doctor. On the part of the doctor, this corresponds to a prayerful relationship with God, Who may grant him the ultimate success of his professional work, which is something outside the doctor's power and which also means that he must assume his professional responsibility in the name of his trust in God. None of the factors mentioned should be neglected. Anyone who wanted to deal only with God would despise both created nature with its remedies and created man with his art, which would be unreligious. And anyone who did not want to go any farther than trusting the doctor would misunderstand the comprehensive reality and significance of his illness.

Patients' expectations can be very different. First there is the health insurance patient who has a completely plain expectation: the doctor is someone who will know his case and can make him well. Once he holds his medicine bottle in his hand, he no longer thinks about the doctor. But such extreme cases are the exception. Another person comes with the same ailment because he has heard of this doctor's reputation. An acquaintance has praised him, was cured by him. Thus the patient has an advance trust that forms the beginning of a personal bond, but also of increased responsibility on the part of the doctor.

A third person has already been successfully treated by this doctor and therefore returns to him with increased trust, perhaps having already recommended him to several others. The doctor will then treat him, no longer as a mere "case", but as an acquaintance, and his treatment will relate to the patient's whole existence.

It happens that a wide variety of patients talk about the doctor in the waiting room and assure each other how highly they regard him. Subsequently, even a kind of collective augmentation can be expected; in a sense, it comes to a kind of creation of the doctor by the patients. The doctor cannot simply remain indifferent to this ideal image, but must try to live up to what is true about it. The patient's expectation may seem to refer to magical powers in the doctor, but the truth behind this appearance is that he is looking for something in the doctor that concerns his whole life, something healing. Patients are often unable to articulate this. They want comfort, advice for special situations, and often they ask in such a way that they already know the answer they want to hear in advance. Of course, one can then treat them according to their superficial mode and give them the answer they already know. In that case, of course, the doctor is in danger of forgetting his responsibility. He simply agrees with the patient, tells him what makes him happy. If he has no worldview himself, the scope of such agreement will be very broad. If he has one, he will perhaps review his answers at the end of a consultation and ponder their moral implications in order to feel his way back to that answer from which all individual answers could be justified, to that overall truth from which all individual truths that he uttered received their legitimacy.

This last point becomes particularly relevant when the patient is struck by severe blows of fate or is about to die. There is nothing more to be done here with mere technology, and the doctor cannot escape, either. He finds himself confronted with the truth about life and death, with God. Even if a patient leaves him, he will have to ask himself whether he did not treat him in a manner all too technical, not holistic enough. In such a situation, the doctor becomes God's patient. He must try to allow himself to be shaped by God. Under no circumstances should he regard his relationship with God as a ready-made recipe and recommend it as such to others, but should expose himself to God's work in order to be able to pass on a living testimony of God.

The doctor's responsibility, which is imposed on him by the patients, is a lonely one. In conversation with them, he must never go so far as to talk to them about their case as with an equal partner. They lack the comprehension of the correlations as he sees them. It is a kind of courtesy on the part of the doctor if he reveals some of his thoughts to them. But he alone is the one ultimately responsible.

If today the cry for patients to have a say is becoming louder and louder, it represents a misjudgment of the facts. The patient can never have the grasp that the doctor has acquired through his studies and practice.

Influence of the Doctor's Worldview

If the doctor has a worldview that for him seems to contain something of the truth of the world, the truth per se, then this worldview must influence all his actions: his relationship with the patient, the recognition of his illness, the measures he takes. It is the primary thing; everything must conform to it and has legitimacy insomuch as it can be integrated into it. Where this is not possible, there must be an error somewhere. If the doctor is consistent in this, he will be increasingly amazed that really nothing of what concerns him lies outside this truth.

Without being asked, he will not tell his patient about his own faith and its mysteries. But the patient will nevertheless realize that, if he confides in the doctor, he will somehow unintentionally come under the law of this truth, even though its law need not affect his own views. If he allows himself to be treated by a Catholic doctor, he may notice that something Catholic also flows into the treatment, without his becoming a different person than he was before. If he is honest, he will have to admit—so long as his illness was a substantial one—that he has been more deeply affected by the Catholic truth than he first assumed. He will at least deal with certain aspects of Catholicism.

If the patient is already a believer, his faith will be revitalized by the manifold impulses experienced during treatment and henceforth occupy a greater space in his existence than before. The illness has also disposed him to think; it is indeed possible that it will take second place for him and the religious question first. A re-evaluation has taken place, which must now also be perceived by the doctor and which requires his constant alertness, since he has become a kind of life-companion. He becomes jointly responsible for the patient's world view. He can certainly give him hints as to how he should evaluate his illness, how he can make it fruitful or come out of it, if it is short-termed, without forgetting, however, certain insights gained from it; and how, on the other hand, he can build himself up toward genuine indifference if the illness is long-termed or terminal.

Approaches to the Church

A lot of people come to the consultations who are ultimately concerned, not with the minor ailment they present to the doctor, but with their life problems. Some tell the doctor all their sins. Others come searching, weighed down by a stifling guilt. Very often it is about marital problems: people have been divorced two or three times, and yet again things don't work out. Where should one go with one's malaise if not to the doctor? He has to deal with all the questions and yet realizes that he is not the right authority. People are in the wrong place: they should actually go to confession. They need to speak out, to be sure, but not only in a psychological sense; mere reassurances will not fix anything. They recognize evil by its consequences, but it should be recognized in its origin. What they need is a forgiveness that no one but God can give, but that the priest can impart: absolution. As a doctor, one necessarily fails here.

The young people come with their problems: premarital sex? Here, too, a Church order stands against a disorder outside of it. The rigidity, the antiquated nature of this order is pointed out from all sides. Rightly so? On the other hand, the doctor is aware of the Church's ban on divorce, which becomes more and more concrete for him in the course of his practice. He sees that the Catholic Church is demanding something objectively correct here that other Christian churches and atheism no longer recognize.

The doctor is directed to the existence of the Church from various sides, perhaps most strongly from patients in their fertile decades. But ultimately the questions cover the entire life from birth to death. Thus the non-Catholic doctor initially has a very schematic image of the Church: her laws are only seen from the outside. But this image demands that one continues to deal with it, until the Church reveals her inner connection with God. From the ban on abortion, the path must be traceable back to God. There must be a line leading from the confession of sin—one without any real distinction between good and evil—back to God's goodness. Then the image of the Church becomes more concrete. One recognizes that one of her hands is in the hand of God, the other in that of the sinner; she is a mediator. And through this concrete mediation, God Himself becomes interesting; He loses his abstractness. In the end, He is not just an object of a recognition, but also a demand on me.

The doctor comes to deal with the Church through his patients, and in order to understand the Church, he would have to get involved with God. What he can impart to his patients, he must first have received himself.

Here he also comes up against a boundary: the priestly office.

The Doctor and the Priest

The doctor is aware that he must not usurp the entire guidance of the patient's soul. If he is a believer and in touch with a priest, cooperation with that priest can be highly fruitful, provided that the patient also belongs to the Church and, if he was alienated from her, can be brought back to her. If both doctor and priest are dependent on each other, with the priest hoping to learn from the doctor the diagnosis and prognosis as well as the overall attitude of the patient and the doctor being cognizant of where the priest's authority begins, and if their cooperation is therefore fruitful for the patient, the patient must not have the feeling that his personal concerns are a topic of conversation between doctor and priest. He remains a free person with his intimacy with God. A great deal of tact is required on the part of both doctor and priest in this respect since the patient has to some extent become the responsibility of both.

Doctor and priest should not only contact each other in extreme cases, but rather, through regular interaction, get a better understanding where their lines of work intersect and try to make the tension between their competences ever more fruitful: for the benefit of the patient as well as for the spreading of the right ecclesial spirit, especially in the hospital. Something like this could have much greater impact than a lot of priestly social work in the parish. If the priest spent more time in the places where the sick are, his influence could be deeper and longer-lasting. If there is a sick person in a family, the family is always broken up, and very often it is open to Christian influence. If it consists of only healthy people, it often appears like a fortress to the outside world.

In view of the priestly authority, the doctor becomes even more aware of his limitations. Even if countless confessions are made during his consultations, often when girls come to find out if they are pregnant and then tell their whole relationship, accusing and justifying themselves at the same time, or when women face an unwanted birth and put the blame on the man and the circumstances, or when people fear that they have contracted a venereal disease, etc., the doctor can do nothing more than give advice. He cannot even demand genuine remorse. Thus, he usually learns that the personal relationship established by the patient does in reality not fully exist. The patient "confesses" because he *must*. But the doctor fails because he *cannot* absolve. This virtually forces him to deal with sacramental confession. There, confession is made out of remorse; here, in the consulting room, it is made out of fear. Absolution by the priest brings the sinner back to God renewed: he is released into the hands of God as a guiltless person. In the case of the patient's confession, there is only the acknowledgment by the doctor, who releases him back into his everyday life. If from then on he is careful not to fall back into sin, it is mainly to avoid the unpleasant situation in the doctor's office. In such a situation, the doctor will, wherever possible, point away from himself to the priest.

But there are also cases when doctors are only too happy to send a patient to the priest. However, this should not be done at the expense of their medical duty. Sin and illness can often be mixed with each other; what constitutes illness is still the responsibility of the doctor. Again, cooperation, where possible, is the best way forward.

Finally, in the case of certain obdurate sinners, the doctor can do some preparatory work for the encounter with the priest: as a Christian, he will not regard and treat any underlying responsibility for the illness as a mere accident, but will try to show it to the patient in its true light. He will not accuse, but talk to the patient so seriously that the patient learns something essential—perhaps new to him—that will have him concerned. When young girls come to the doctor to find out if they are pregnant, it is almost always possible to open up a real conversation. And because the doctor is the last and only person of respect for many of them, he can also share some of his own views. He can explain his reasons for rejecting extramarital intercourse and show why they should not be trivialized. This attitude of not taking sin for granted provides the doctor with a large target area, and patients are usually more receptive to this than one might think.

A Book by Paul Tournier[2]

Paul Tournier's first book, *Médecine de la Personne*,[3] had an unexpectedly inspiring effect on many lay people,

[2] Dr. Paul Tournier, *De la Solitude à la Communauté* (Delachaux et Niéstlé, 1943).

[3] English title: *The Healing of Persons*, trans. Edwin Hudson (Harper and Row, 1965).

doctors, and clergy. For the first time, a doctor so openly confessed that he was nothing more than an instrument in God's hands and that his own knowledge and skills would remain ineffective as long as the patient did not entrust himself and his illness to God. The doctor may well take all those measures for the detection and healing of suffering that correspond to the state of his science, but for the main thing, for the recovery of the soul and the resolution of all conflicts that both daily life and illness bring with them, he plays no other role than that of a guide who tirelessly points in the same direction: to the path to God.

The book was written entirely in the spirit of the Oxford Movement and was bound to inspire completely its followers above all; but it could also give valuable pointers to religious seekers who are entangled in their personal difficulties and see no way out; indeed, it described so many individual cases that almost everyone could recognize himself or at least part of himself and his experiences in the book.

A second book by Tournier has recently been published: *De la Solitude à la Communauté*.[4] In it, we encounter essentially the same problems, which are discussed using concrete examples from practice. The people we encounter here still bring the same problems to the doctor, their lack of redemption in the midst of their daily mistakes and sins; and using the

[4] English title: *Escape from Loneliness*, trans. John S. Gilmour (John Knox, 1977).

same method, communal prayer, the doctor tries to convey to them the healing that lies in the encounter with God. In view of this method, and given its exclusivity, the question arises for the Catholic doctor and patient: To what extent can we agree with it and even imitate it, and to what extent must we decisively distance ourselves from it?

The patients in Tournier's second book are almost entirely lonely people who are tormented by their loneliness and whose illness consists more in a general unease toward life than in a precisely definable clinical picture. In conventional medical terms, they would be more in need of psychiatric counseling. The appealing thing about Tournier is that he departs from conventional psychology and psychiatry; he wants nothing to do with this dissection of the soul that penetrates to the deepest spiritual secrets in order to lift them out individually, solve them, and assemble them into a new whole according to a specific plan. As a Christian, he knows that such an action is basically unreligious, even impossible, because the soul has its most hidden foundation in God Himself, in a region where no healing science—which only knows about clinical pictures and medical measures—can ever reach. The soul belongs to its Creator; He alone can work the ultimate in it. The doctor can at best indicate certain points, uncover them in love, but the patient must learn to realize that the heaviness that weighs on him is his sin, which not the doctor but God alone can lift away from him. He must learn that God's grace alone can help him and that his sin is the obstacle to experiencing God's love for him as well as his own love for God.

All of this is excellent. The worrisome part begins when the doctor tries to treat the effect of God like a medication, dosing it almost like an injection and thus degrading the greatness of God, Who remains intrinsically unpredictable in His work, to a factor in his small medical healing plan. Loving God and knowing Him does not mean having the power to summon Him at any time as needed; nowhere is tact more imperative than in religious intimacy. God certainly leaves to the sinner's soul, which He claims for Himself, its independence; He even increases it, but He also reserves His own; for if our attachment to God ultimately means freedom, then even more so His attachment to us. If man's love for God is expressed in the words "Thy will be done", then this will usually has a different form from what our earthly thinking expects. The prayer of the Oxfordian, however, seems more or less clearly to carry within itself the right to a certain fulfillment, thus making God a function of one's own will. We take offense at this. We are convinced that God answers every prayer, but this answer need by no means become apparent to us, especially not apparent in the sense we ourselves desire.

Of course, the author is far from using faith and religion—as certain psychiatrists like to do—as a proven remedy for specific and special categories of mental illnesses, while other illnesses require a different treatment. God, in Tournier's system, is a remedy in a far more subtle and beautiful sense. And yet our discomfort with his method remains—precisely because it is a method. In the second book, this seems to intensify, the author seems to have tightened his expectations and modified his method for the purpose of simplification, almost for a recipe that is as uncomplicated as possible. A certain schematization (not to say mechanization) of the external framework and the act itself seems to have occurred. The interspersed philosophical digressions are unable to dispel this impression of impoverishment, because the author's talent does not lie in philosophy; his explanations at this point are rather nebulous and cannot be rounded into a whole. They contribute nothing to a deeper understanding of the basic idea. Let us add that the lack of humor and the utter non-musicality of expression make the book even more difficult to read. Despite occasionally concise formulations, Tournier is not a writer and the laboriousness of his compilations is all too evident. As a result, the author's enjoyment of his work seems somewhat colorless for the most part; it is exhausted in itself, as it were, and therefore lacks the power of contagion with the reader. Perhaps this is also due to the fact that the personality of the doctor is too much in the foreground, although the author knows and emphasizes that his effect should be purely instrumental and thus comparable to the effect of the saints, who radiate what they have received from God and thereby make it easier for people to find their way to God. Precisely because Tournier speaks so positively of some

Catholic saints, the distance between his thoughts and their intentions and aspirations becomes palpable. For not only do they possess to a perfect degree the art of diminishing before God, to Whom they point, they also know above all that the ways of God can never be systematically determined.

In the medical field, we are already familiar with a wide variety of issues, diagnostic methods, healing procedures, etc. It would never do to want to treat everything with a single prescription, a limited healing method. Tournier is also concerned with healing; indeed, his field, which lies in the spiritual-religious, is decidedly even more differentiated than the physical. Is it acceptable to limit the treatment here to a single "spiritual experience", that of the confession of sin? In view of the infinite differentiation of souls and destinies by God, how can this concise, almost tediously simple method not impair, indeed, unconsciously abandon, the fullness of divine possibilities, how can this monotonous formula not kill all the riches of grace and degrade God to the owner of a meager mechanism, while man becomes an almost meaningless shell that only needs to turn its inside out—and perhaps not even necessarily toward God—in order to get rid of its worries and obtain a worldly successful and (what is worse) Christianly satisfied life in return?

The patient who goes to Tournier knows quite accurately what awaits him in advance. He will confess his sins, the doctor will pray with him, and the sufferer will record what God subscribes for him in a kind of inner vision—the nature of which remains obscure to us. He will then compare it with the doctor's notes, the latter will discuss the result, and thus the healing is initiated. Here, too, it is clear that the expectation—both before and after the consultation—is a very specific one. If the element of surprise is thus removed, the emotional readiness eases the heaviness of the confession; the patient has already come to terms with it before going to the doctor, he is therefore already willing to undertake the joint prayer: he is already on the way to recovery.

In this respect, the Oxfordian confession of sin has much in common with the Catholic confession. And yet the differences are more profound than the similarities. To say nothing of others: once God has forgiven the confessing Catholic, the matter is closed for him, he no longer talks about it, he begins to live as a new person, which does not mean at all that he will not succumb to the same mistakes again. But the sins committed and confessed are completely erased by the grace of God. With the Oxfordians, on the other hand, the sin remains at the center of further proceedings; although one is detached from it through the public confession—perhaps precisely because of this—one returns to it again and again; one speaks of it at every opportunity, lets it shine in its demonic splendor; it becomes, because it is now public, the core of conversion; without it, the sinner would never have come to God; over time it acquires the character of a kind of sanctuary. While all the light thus shines on the moment of conversion, the further fate of the sinner himself remains rather vague. But it seems to be thought of in analogy to those infectious diseases that one only goes through once and then remains permanently immune to. There are certainly mistakes that can be avoided in the future. But aren't they the exceptions? And if, after serious illness, certain foods or efforts cause relapses, can all temptations that will necessarily arise again after serious sin be overcome with such ease that—as the book implies—there is no need to speak of them at all? Is there not a danger of Pharisaism here, both in the assumption that sin will no longer be committed in the future and in measuring oneself against the greatness of one's own sin, whose main characteristic remains that it was committed before the conversion? The most that can be said is that God redeems Christianity *because* of its sin, but he always redeems the individual *despite* his sin.

Conversion is never an act completed once and for all, never an isolated, measurable event. It is a real movement. This movement takes time to unfold, a great deal of time, in fact. Very rarely can one expect instantaneous changes that become outwardly apparent. What grows all too quickly remains premature and soon decays; the true recovery after serious illness is the slow one. In order for strength to be sufficient for a normal life, it must first be regained. From Tournier's patients, however, we generally only learn about the medical history until the change for the better; nothing more after that. It is as if the advertised remedy can help to overcome a crisis, but we do not learn whether it proves just as effective in the subsequent crises that are sure to occur. Tournier's entire relationship with his patients is a beginning that can be suitable in individual cases to lead from the impersonal coolness of Protestantism into a warmer atmosphere and thus awaken a feeling of security in the sick person. But this beginning should turn into a lasting movement.

Tournier is undoubtedly a courageous Christian; his life and his books prove it. We are deeply indebted to his Christian commitment, despite all the criticism of the shortcomings of his confession, which has become a method. His suggestions have the allure of the new; perhaps they will also achieve the duration of the true, which would be possible if they no longer intertwined grace and psychology, sacrament and analysis. For Catholics, this would mean close cooperation between doctor and priest in the peripheral areas between medicine and pastoral care, without allowing the two disciplines to coincide. Finally, even the so-called healthy could learn from Tournier and his patients that, in addition to illness and sorrow, one can and should leave one's health, happiness, and all pleasures up to God, and finally one's entire existence, so as to leave it in His hands and live entirely according to His pleasing.

A Selection from a Novel by Gotthelf[5]

Through her birth, Anne Bäbi Jowäger revolutionizes all our views on the possibilities of conception, for she was created by a decree of the Bernese authorities in the imagination of a poet. The other medical problems she addresses, however, are quite modern, so much so that one cannot tell they are from a hundred years ago. Even today, doctors come across them every day. In her abundant considerations, Anne Bäbi sees herself as quite an expert, and not just in one special field of medicine, but practically in all of them; she knows in advance what will do good and what will not. She draws this knowledge from the treasure trove of her human experience and always comes to the conclusion, which is never fully formulated, yet shines through everywhere, that it is not the medicine that matters, but the doctor, his personality. Since she herself is a differentiated thinker, her own substitution of the doctor seems easy to her. She is happy to take his place in a small circle and would have no objection if the number of people seeking advice from her were to increase.

Anne Bäbi quite rightly distinguishes between prevention and cure. When it comes to prevention, she

[5] The fragment from the novel is written in Bernese dialect, which renders the narrative more colorful and makes the character of Anne Bäbi more tangible. It is impossible to do the dialect justice in English.—Trans.

knows that it is best to avoid sin, although her concept of sin is subject to all sorts of fluctuations. For her, not sinning means, above all, not doing anything that could humiliate her in her own eyes or diminish her material prestige in any way. She believes that her prosperity is reflected above all in her food, and since her medical care is devoted first and foremost to her late-born only son Jakobli,[6] he must remain healthy especially through food.

> A slice of meat would do a child particular good, said Anne Bäbi. Nothing makes the flesh as healthy as meat does, especially if it was in the smoking chamber for a while. So said Anne Bäbi, and if an angel had come from heaven and said: "Listen, Anne Bäbi, the good Lord sends you his greetings and tells you that the cream is too fattening for your little boy, the meat is too spicy for your little boy, that's where his bad ears and eyes come from, milk is more than enough, even if you were to add some water to it, it wouldn't do any harm, and he could probably use a slice of fresh meat, but no other," Anne Bäbi would have continued with cream and bacon and thought to herself: "The good Lord doesn't understand this; in heaven you wouldn't know what cream and bacon could do, and what you don't understand, in God's name you shouldn't meddle with."[7]

[6] The *-li* is a diminutive. The effect is akin to *Li'l Jacob*.—TRANS.

[7] Jeremias Gotthelf, *Anne Bäbi Jowäger*, vol. 1 (Birkhäuser, 1949), 14.

So Anne Bäbi would not shy away from giving explanations to the good Lord so that he would be able to revise some of his views. And yet she remains faithful to the idea that illness and sin are closely linked. The difference to Tournier's views is perhaps not very significant, although the connections are not exactly close: Anne Bäbi wants to prevent illness from arising in the first place by abstaining from sin, whereas Tournier seeks above all to cure illness by turning away from sin.

Only the obvious is suitable to make Anne Bäbi think more deeply; this thinking, however, she does thoroughly and gives it her entire character. She works out the laws of guilt and atonement very carefully, but in such a way that she has nothing to do with them personally, yet believes she has the knowledge to draw the right conclusions for others, such as her dear neighbors. She draws the abundance of her axioms from the depths of her inner being and only accepts the experiences of others if they help her to regain seemingly lost ground while saving her own reputation, which ultimately remains her highest priority. The good Lord, who somehow lurks in the background, takes on a very strange form, because He consists largely of an accumulation of arguments that she has crafted herself, only to bring them out at the right moment, adorned with the necessary complementary colors. In this, Anne Bäbi embodies a mentality that is still quite relevant today. If we excerpt what she knows about the nature of illness, about its development or prevention, we can easily see that all of it still lives on happily today, that the multicolored nature of her theory and insights has lost none of its power. To encounter them all, more or less clearly, in their own originality, one need only venture a walk into the vicinity of our hospitals, at the time when the flood of visitors is pouring out . . .

Present the development of medicine in such a way that one realizes: everything bears the stamp of the provisional. But the character of man is not provisional. Develop the doctor-patient relationship from that. This relationship bears the same characteristics as in Anne Bäbi's time. Medicine would perhaps gain a definitive direction if this relationship gained a living direction.

Since Anne Bäbi knows better than God, she naturally knows everything better than the doctor from the outset. The trust-relationship with the doctor could and should be developed into a trust-relationship with God.

The Doctor's Prayer and Contemplation

Perhaps more than anyone else, a doctor is constantly called upon to recognize his own limitations. With every serious surgery and every unexpected incident, he comes up against them. And every time a difficult case ends well, he feels relieved. Upon closer consideration, he feels that a particular fortune has favored him. In cases that end badly, however, while he had a better prognosis, he cannot shake off the feeling that he has made a mistake somewhere. Nevertheless, if he remains objective when reconstructing the whole case, he has to admit to himself that he probably did everything that was medically necessary. In this constant oscillation between "fortune" and "misfortune", he often runs the risk of becoming *superstitious*, because he has to ascribe a secret role to something that is not his own doing and yet is somehow involved. There is a large number of doctors who have no faith but, instead, a considerable dose of superstition. They would never start a risky operation with a knife that has already been used, would not operate on a Friday unless it was urgent, would take special care with the third operation, would not bring a seriously ill new patient into a room where someone had just died, etc. Such a doctor has the feeling that he is dealing with forces that he cannot conquer, and he grants these alleged forces considerable leeway.

For the doctor, on the other hand, who possesses genuine faith, it is certain that where *life* is at stake, where important surgeries are concerned or where unforeseen "coincidences" (in the medical sense) occur, it cannot just be a question of a struggle between his skills and the illness, but must be a confrontation of his whole being with the life of the patient, in a commitment that he somehow dares to make, that seems justified to him on the basis of his knowledge and experience and the current state of medicine, but in which an entire realm is left to God. If he realizes this, he would probably have to give greater importance to prayer in his life. Before every important surgery, before every encounter, he would then commend his patient and his medical plan to God. Perhaps he would do this in the manner of people who begin to pray when they feel attacked or are particularly afflicted by grief and suffering, but then forget about praying again in everyday life. Accordingly, a doctor who does not really *live* by faith will likewise pray much less when it comes to everyday encounters.

But perhaps he will have bad luck in a case where he did not pray. Then he may become aware of an omission. Or he may be lucky in the very place where he did pray and could now get the feeling of being able to count on God. Then he, too, would be close to superstition. But if he gives himself an account of what prayer really should be, then it should become clear to him that it must not be a mere act on the spur of the moment, that we should not only call upon God when we ourselves can no longer cope, but rather that God's Son became man in order to share our whole life, not just its exciting events, but everyday life, and that His relationship with us in his earthly life was a reliable one. He has persevered with us in all our life situations, even where no one thought it necessary to seek Him out.

Now the doctor realizes that his prayer must not be left to chance; rather, he must enter into a relationship with God that possesses the duration and perseverance desired and given by God Himself; indeed, he should try to lead a life in God, a life of prayer. His prayer will then take on a new form. This will not prevent him from counting on God's help especially in moments of danger, but on the help of a God *who is there*, whose demands he knows, indeed, with whom he is actually in constant conversation. It certainly cannot be a matter of the doctor outwardly acting as a prayerful person and thus taking on the role of the priest. But neither can it be a matter of having a secret religion, of regarding one's conversation with God as a purely private matter between oneself and God and of approaching people with an attitude in which no effect of this conversation can be felt. There is no rule for how to observe the golden mean, but there is an overall attitude that points to God, even if the name of God is rarely mentioned, an attitude that is Christian and ecclesiastical, that instills trust in the patient, that not only relates to the person treating him, but constantly points him to the One Who also guides the doctor's life.

By repeatedly presenting their problems to the doctor for a solution, patients continuously give him material for *contemplation*. And because his contemplation focuses not only on the illness, but above all on the sick person, it becomes a matter of *charity*. But because this is a part of the love of God and is encompassed in it, the doctor's contemplation of the patient's problems cannot be detached from the questions that God asks of man in general. In this way, the contemplation of our fellow man is expanded and finds its place in the contemplation of God, while the contemplation of God always leads back to our sick fellow men without ever becoming one-sided. After all, there is nothing in the fullness of what Christ reveals to us that does not also have its place in the problems of our fellow men, just as, conversely, God's truths already emerge in the midst of our own problems.

On the other hand, the doctor's contemplation must not have such a vaguely general character that it ultimately no longer relates to anything in particular. Like every Christian, he should set aside times in his daily work that are reserved for explicit prayer, and from there allow it to illuminate the rest of the day. All forms of prayer are available to him, personal and ecclesiastical, spoken and contemplative; and just as he does not commit himself to a single method in his medical methodology, he will also try to test the diversity of Christian prayer in his prayer life. If he sets up a program for himself and sticks to its baselines, he will certainly not exclude anything that can enrich this program. Just as he is prepared constantly to expand his medical knowledge through study and experience, he will also try constantly to expand his prayer through contemplation and reading and make it livelier.

But he must not become an itinerant preacher and sectarian. He should work more through his attitude than through the direct word, imitate the Lord more where He is the Logos according to His essence, rather than where He is the Logos in His spoken word. The doctor will not talk much about God, but rather answer to the patient's concrete questions and needs.

It is also the case that the doctor must constantly *demand* things from the patient. He gives him measures, prescriptions, orders, and expects them to be followed. In this expectation lies the possibility for him to teach the patient *obedience*. This is by no means a matter of course. Among his patients, there are many who, as much as possible, are used to doing only what they like. In order to know how his demands affect the patient, what powers are at the patient's disposal in order to be obedient, the doctor must have tested and acquired these powers in himself, let them work in himself, *live* from them. A doctor who knows only his own good judgment as a rule, who acts only according to the inspiration of the moment, and with a large dose of *know-it-all attitude*, cannot demand obedience. He should behave as seriously with regard to the commandments of life, the demands of God, as he expects the patient to behave with regard to his instructions.

The Sick Doctor

Like anyone else, a sick doctor may, according to his temperament, either trivialize his illness and from the outset consider only a good outcome possible, or, on the contrary, see everything black in black, exaggerate all symptoms and make the most pessimistic diagnoses. But one thing is certain: symptoms that you experience yourself look different from those that you only know from patients' descriptions. You have imagined everything with different nuances. If it is more than just a little flu, even the sick doctor will eventually go to the doctor—not without presuppositions, but burdened with his medical experience and with all the more or less correct conclusions he has drawn in advance about his illness. He usually expects his own diagnosis to be confirmed; he does not realize how difficult it is to experience things from the inside that one is used to looking at from the outside. But what he experiences, he must now come to terms with. His medical history—if it is a real illness—generally seems much more special to him, much more original than that of other people. Perhaps rightly so, inasmuch as introspection is part of his profession somewhere: if he already has a picture of the illness he is experiencing, the individual symptoms are more distinctive for him than for an ordinary patient who has no idea of what is part of this clinical picture.

He also has a certain opinion of his colleague's skills. He has chosen *this* particular colleague because he values his competence from experience. Something objective is reflected in this, which, however, blends with something subjective: if he now becomes a patient of this colleague, he likes to set his expectations so high that disappointment is inevitable. For the doctor who has to treat a doctor, the difficulties are not small. Firstly because the patient comes with many medical presuppositions and is more or less fixed on his own diagnosis and the measures to be taken, and secondly because the attending doctor sees his colleague in the patient and feels somehow exposed by him. Things that he normally diagnoses without difficulty and carries out with certainty, since he assumes that the patient accepts them as proven, strangely lose their evidence and their luster. He expects confirmation from his sick colleague. If he receives it, he is nevertheless never quite sure whether he has acted correctly, or whether the other person has not agreed out of tiredness or politeness. He also knows that the colleague has described his symptoms to him through a doctor's temperament, somehow already stylized toward the diagnosis. All this explains why doctors are so difficult to treat and why there is so much mishap between doctors. Doctors are very often treated incorrectly.

The doctor must be able to approach his patient freely. There are prerequisites for the functioning of a doctor's intuition. Because of my daily consultation hours, I am always used to being the knowing one to the unknowing. Even if I am convinced that I don't know everything and am a little skeptical about my skills, I do acquire a certain degree of certainty over time. My honesty makes me vigilant at best, not insecure. Even in a doctor who has nothing to do with quackery and who sincerely endeavors to proceed scientifically, the human element plays such a large role that his technique is, as it were, enveloped by the human element: by his human certainty and his will to help. Even the safest scientific skill has a personal imprint.

Therefore, where something serious is at stake, the attending doctor should demand from the sick doctor the liberty to face him only as a physician faces a patient and to be allowed to give his instructions as he would to any other patient. For his part, the patient should try not to feel like a doctor during the course of his illness, not to hinder the attending doctor with his own views and wishes. He should not tempt him to act as he himself would have acted in the same case, as this only causes mutual confusion.

This makes it clear to the attending doctor that he has to treat each patient anonymously, as it were, even though the doctor loves him and wants to support him. That he has a right to treat everyone as he seriously believes to be right. He should maintain a kind of objectivity toward every patient, but at the same time this objectivity is so rooted in the human and ideological that every relationship with every patient is ultimately the same and lives from the same power. If the sick doctor is honest enough to admit this to himself, he knows that only under such conditions one can work uninhibitedly; he will avoid everything that inhibits the other person. He will trust him as he would like every patient to trust himself. If he has difficulty in accepting the role of the mere patient, then he should consider what he himself demands of his patients. His own difficulty gives him an understanding of his patients' difficulties. If he overcomes them, he learns to help them overcome them as well. In this way, his illness can become just as much a new beginning for him as his former studies. His experiences are reorganized from a different perspective.

The Doctor and Christ

The Christian doctor knows that he must draw the strength to exercise his daily profession as a vocation from God. For he does not possess it once and for all, as one possesses one's nature, but as something that even though it is always available, must always be asked for anew.

God is also behind the natural realm. He gives the physician his knowledge. God has hidden many secrets in nature, not forbidding us to explore them, but in tension with the talent of man, who is to explore and gratefully appropriate them. God wants this struggle of man with nature, and also the struggle of the doctor with illness; for this purpose, God has given him a certain superiority that is an image and likeness of His divine superiority.

Whereas God still remains half concealed in these relationships with nature, He reveals Himself in the Gospel, where His Son deals with people on earth, which actually takes place consistently under the parable of the physician. For people, says Jesus, are sick people who need a physician; and those who think they are healthy need him the most. Thus not only the scenes in which He explicitly heals the sick or raises the dead bear witness to His work, but also all those in which He forgives sins and endeavors to heal people's souls. He conveys this health with His full commitment. Significantly, when He heals the woman with the issue of blood, He says He perceives that power has gone forth from Him.

His healing miracles are "signs"; they are images, reminders of the deeper healing of the whole person. But these signs are not indifferent to the deeper dimension, because the Word really has become flesh; through His flesh, It redeems us on the Cross. This is why the bodily signs have something sacramental about them. For the Son, His Father's creation is not something neutral that is subordinate to Him. He often uses it as a remedy in His healing miracles. He moistens the eyes of a blind man with saliva or prepares a kind of dirt from street dust and saliva, which He spreads on the eyes of the sick person. He instructs His disciples to anoint the suffering with oil and so on. When John the Baptist asks Him whether He is the Messiah, He answers by pointing out that the blind see, the lame walk, the lepers are cleansed and the dead are raised. That is how important these signs seem to Him.

Of course, the Son of God does not come as an earthly doctor. He does not build hospitals. He wants to heal man as a whole, that is, to make him fit for God. But He also uses bodily healing for this purpose, and as a result the art of medicine takes on a whole new significance. If medicine, practiced within the realm of creation, seems to belong somehow to the Old Testament—a kind of equalizer of justice—then in the New Testament it becomes a function of the love that gratefully makes use of all the possibilities given to it by God, and these possibilities go beyond the purely natural. Not as if man should not also make progress in science; God wants this, and mere conservatism would be ingratitude to the Creator. God demands a kind of progress that deserves its name in God's sense, while any progress that deviates from God's intentions does not deserve its name in a Christian sense. But the love of Christ goes far beyond the natural sphere, which is why medical practice in His succession will have to follow in this transition. Christ thinks of the glorification of the Father in everything. The proper doctor must do the same and be careful not to practice his craft in unbelief. (Ultimately, there is no neutral medicine: it works toward God or against Him.)

The doctor knows that he cannot compete with Christ. He is not a savior. But if he believes that the power of the Lord is as alive among us today as it was then, indeed that this power is made available to people even more than it was then, then he can ask from this power what he needs for his work as a follower of Christ. He remains aware of the distance; he will not want to conduct his conversations with patients according to the Lord's words in the Gospel or perform healing miracles solely on the basis of his faith. He has to radiate the disposition of Christ within his field, nothing more.

In one respect, he will imitate the example of Christ: every person He meets He takes personally and treats accordingly. He has no general recipe. He only pays attention to one thing: how He can simultaneously carry out the will of the Father in this encounter and touch the innermost being of the person standing before Him. The doctor should not act in a stereotypical manner, either, but should besides his knowledge also consult the richness of his faith, the fullness of which protects him from any sterility in his professional actions.

By sending illness to a person, God intervenes in his personal life and sets a reminder of his creation and mortality. The sick person, deprived of his busyness, cannot help but think of the last things. And through the healing, God can once again speak another word to him, make clear to him something of His power to bestow rebirth. Beyond all scientifically recognizable laws of regeneration, through the illness and its healing, patient and doctor are reminded of the ultimate cause. But the "God factor" must not be counted by the doctor as one among others in the healing process—that is Tournier's mistake—just as Christ always behaved in a new and different way in his encounters with sinners and the sick, so will God show Himself in a new way in every relationship between doctor and patient.

The Father is glorified in Christ's miraculous healings. Not only through the miracle as such, but just as much through the healing. The person concerned lives ten years longer, in accordance with the will of the Father, and the Son has submitted to this will. Analogously, the doctor works to ensure that a person remains alive until the date appointed by God. Certainly the doctor does not know this date; when he heals a seriously ill, perhaps dying person, it looks as if God places this date in his hands. Looking deeper, this remains a mystery between God and the Christian who believes in Him. Of course, the unbeliever can come along and say that an unbelieving doctor with the same skill could have achieved the same results. But this objection does not hold water when you consider that the duration of every life ultimately depends on God's predestination. The unbelieving doctor is only a planned episode in it; it is not he to whom God gives the gift of the patient's life. God allows the healing to succeed so that the patient can thank God and the doctor has yet another opportunity to think of God. With the believing doctor, the relationship is different: God not only gives him the gift of the patient's life, he also lets him give the gift. Ultimately, the truly gifted person is the believing doctor, who is gifted by God through the gift he gives to God.

V

SCATTERED NOTES

Won't the moment come for you when, with God's help, you learn to bear the thought of death, the thought of your illness lasting until death? Is it not better for you to bear precisely what God gives you? Don't you want to be like healthy people at least in this respect, that you remain on the path of God, as He now demands of you? Your illness hardly gives you the right to turn away from God in order to go your own ways.

And if your illness is such that you can count on recovery, then at least use it as a time of reflection. Gather experiences that to you, and even more so to those around you, can be valuable later.

The patient as a critical case: educate him about it and explain to him the reciprocity of the service (between him and the doctor). Even the student should be aware of this reciprocity. Try to bring the patient closer to him (in human terms): Why not give him the spiritual

The vast majority of these notes are originally in German, but some of them are interspersed with French fragments, others are entirely in French.—Trans.

responsibility for a few beds, a room, so that he may grow into precisely this most important area?

Patient, we call on you to cooperate. The optimistic patient shows much better healing tendencies than the pessimistic one.

The conclusions that the anamnesis alone allows us to draw about the nature, character, and illness of the patient: half of the diagnosis is already made before the patient is examined.

Make an attempt out of my life to give people a life of their own. We want to teach you to suffer pain in all its magnitude, and then you show us how to suffer.

It has always been clear that the embryo possesses a human nature from the beginning. The child has a soul and therefore an inviolable right to life. Therefore, there are no indications for abortion, neither medical nor eugenic nor social. The doctor who decides to perform an abortion degrades himself and transitions from what is his profession—healing—to killing.

By accident, an abortion can be induced without sin: if the abortion is secondary to a cure for a fatal illness of the mother.

Principles:

1. The embryo is not a diseased part of the mother's body, but a human being.
2. The child is never an unjust aggressor.

3. The life of the child is not to be regarded as worthless because it is endangered.

4. The life of the mother is not in itself more precious than that of the child.

5. Most impressive is (the objection): if the child is killed, at least the mother remains alive. But natural death and homicide are two different things.

The Church has never changed her position. Medicine is in a state of development and, like any science, is constantly changing.

Thomas Aquinas (applied to sterilization today): "Never must corporal punishment that consists in killing or mutilation or chastisement be inflicted on an innocent person by a human court." The individual has no right of disposal over the members of his body other than that he may use them according to their natural purpose; he may therefore neither destroy nor mutilate them, nor in any other way render them unfit for their natural functioning, unless the welfare of the body as a whole cannot be otherwise provided for. So says the Christian moral teaching, and the same follows from mere reason.

Does the scope of medical truth coincide with that of the organism? Or does it include things that take place outside the individual human being? Is there a real encounter between the objectivity of a fully grasped medical truth and the objectivity of faith?

The ego of the patient and the ego of the doctor must be objectified, not only by science but by the "Higher Subject".

Proper contemplation is objective in any case.

The encounter of our historicity with the historicity of the patient: the same disease in another age would perhaps show other temporal factors, because the illness is subject to temporal changes. And much more: a doctor from another era would judge differently and take different measures; his personal judgment also remains not only person- but time-dependent.

Very often, genius springs forth from contemplation. The (Christian) contemplative practice has its counterpart in the doctor's intuition, which springs forth from a habit of scientific meditation, whereby knowledge corresponds roughly to faith (irrevocably, irrefutably).

The stories that people tell in the consultation may all be true (somehow), but what work the doctor has to do to glean out of it the truth that alone matters!

A doctor's actions should actually also be a confession. My knowledge reaches this far: I confess it to myself.

Become, for there is no being in us.

The clinician: "Examine." The psychiatrist: "Put yourself in relation." Whereby the psychiatrist's method reveals his own essence.

The patient is a partner and not an object. Science is *only* a foundation; it is *only* at the beginning of its development; it knows successes and failures. Science is therefore nothing final.

Do not by my actions hinder God in his actions.

Dangers for the doctor: no longer increasing the knowledge acquired during studies, simply allowing it to be absorbed into the practitioner's skills. You only ever hear negative things about your colleagues from the patients. Remember that you are sitting in the same glass house.

We know how imprecise we are in our own thinking, how easily we give up a thought when it takes an effort to think it through. And yet our most noble task is to help others to think, for how often does their illness consist mainly of wrong trains of thought (proven by the example of youth enlightenment, non-marriage).

Know how to be sick; teach it to people and learn it from them.

As a doctor, one should be able to endure both frequent successes and failures.

What emerges from the purely rational realm is eminently present in medicine and shapes the doctor.

Prepare the patient's mind just as the body to handle the illness or the surgery.

The doctor and the patient pursue the same goal. The problem of confidence on either side.

Attitude. The relationship between the doctor's attitude and the patient's attitude; their ability to influence one another mutually. To what extent does the urgent need for cooperation depend on attitude? The attitude (of the doctor) is a result dependent on the worldview, the character, the ability, the skills, the knowledge, and the goal to be achieved. The goal of the profession should be reflected in each individual case.

The presence of a patient in the consulting room is the result of an inner attitude that, however, even still in the waiting room is subject to all kinds of fluctuations and can be fundamentally changed by the ambiance or also by the doctor himself. Certainly there are also "good" attitudes that do not require correction; others remain impossible to influence, even though they are harmful and not adapted to the illness.

And if it were God's will for you to have a fatal illness, perhaps the very illness you have been afraid of all your life, you would have to bear and affirm it, and this would by no means be a heroic deed, but an attempt, undertaken in humility, to show God that your faith is a serious reality for you and that you have at least grasped something of his demand in this respect.

Illness means a disturbance of your well-being; the disturbance can be of a very serious nature or hardly worthy of attention; either way, it is a warning, it is meant to remind you of your death, to remind you once and for all that there are limits to your earthly life. You do not need to know where they are, when they will appear to you; you should only keep in mind: they are there. Is this realization not important enough in itself to give your illness of whatever kind its full meaning, to make it appear to you as a time placed at your special disposal? So it has to fulfill its very specific purpose: to make you more familiar with Christ. Your bedridden state, your quiet and seclusion give you the necessary stillness: You can let God work on you; you can listen to Him; you have long hours ahead of you that are not merely filled with everyday silence, perhaps passing in pain, hours that belong to you and are otherwise rarely given to you in this way, to you alone, so that you may use them according to your own choosing, good or bad; you may use them for reflection, for fortifying yourself, but do it with the help of God, give them to Him first, as you give yourself to Him anew. Science and pastoral care: Is it necessary to separate them so fundamentally during your studies that pastoral care not only becomes a *fetus papyraceus*, but remains completely nonexistent?

The Doctor on His Way to God

I made a good diagnosis and the patient recovered. But I had no opportunity to have a proper conversation with him. The opportunity might have presented itself if my own point of view had been different. I only perceived the patient within my limited medical horizon. Something in me says: It is my fault that I did not establish a better relationship with him. But what was lacking in me? Somewhere an certain emptiness remained, especially when things were going very well. I lacked a relationship with God, so I did not get in touch with the patient, either.

The other extreme: I made every conceivable effort, but everything went wrong. The patient died or transferred to another doctor. I cannot bear my failure, neither as a doctor nor as a person. Where should I take this failure? Based on my previous notion of God, certainly not to Him. At best, I could accuse fate or say to God: I have done the best I could. Comfort me! But then I would just fall back on myself. Do I have to change my relationship with God?

A third case: My relationship with a patient was normal throughout the illness. We talked to each other. He showed me that in philosophical terms he was a seeker. I would have liked to show him that I live entirely from God, but I didn't dare. Why not? Because I am still a seeker myself. I would probably have to convert in order to be able to say the crucial word. As long as I seek, I cannot want to lead. Of course, as a doctor you have the right to still have problems, but with certain things you should have come to terms: the ultimate personal questions.

If we propose to live in the truth in medicine, we must submit to the harshest of ethics; its limits are unlimited, for there is not *one* truth, but an incalculable number, many of which fight each other and several of which stifle each other. The center of truth cannot, by definition, be the place where the doctor finds himself; he must be content to live somewhere within a circle of truth, and know that he is off-center.

The truth of my feelings (affection, sympathy) in medical dramas and their contribution of operational medical inefficiency.

Indiscretion and truth have nothing to do with each other. For even where that which should be concealed is expressed, untruth begins: breaching the sacred is already a lie. Professional secrecy means preserving things inside, where they preserve their true cause.

What is truth for the doctor? His philosophy? His own being? The being of the patient? The mutual relationship? As a personal one? Or as that of one who knows to one who confides? The science? The medical skill?

Are the patient's symptoms truth-revealing? But to what extent are they not simultaneously truth-concealing, because diagnostics are not yet sufficiently advanced? Or because it actually creates the patient's personality to a certain extent?

The truth takes on a completely different, subjectively differently graspable character, depending on whether an anonymous illness (but where would this exist?) is looking for an anonymous helper or this particular patient is looking for this particular doctor.

Where understanding ends, gossip begins; when you hear it, you are amazed at the small space that understanding occupies.

Medical truth has no abstract character, but becomes true in the one who experiences it, thus very often independently of the one who reveals, conveys, or confirms it.

Truth is actually only effective when it is—or becomes—the same for both the doctor and the patient.

Truth does not mean healing; it is occasionally responsible for serious damage: suicide after revealing a diagnosis, letting oneself go in the case of incurable illnesses.

There is a negative and a positive fullness of truth.

Truth and uncertainty often go hand in hand in medicine.

Within the same truth, what is the main thing for one person (thus the main truth) is a secondary matter for the other (thus a peripheral truth).

Often the sick person arrives at a proper attitude toward the truth for the first time through his illness and then recognizes the untruth of the previous.

The charismatic gift of healing comes from the Spirit, but the commission (to heal) comes from Christ, the Word that is the Truth.

Objective and subjective in their actual and in their seeming opposition.

On the nonsense of medical science. Is perfect comprehensibility desirable if through the refinement of the methodology in the examinations the man is taken farther away from us?